THE
SWITCH

THE
SWITCH

IGNITE YOUR METABOLISM WITH INTERMITTENT
FASTING, PROTEIN CYCLING, AND KETO

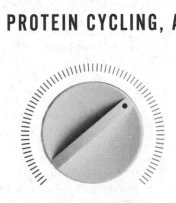

JAMES W. CLEMENT

WITH KRISTIN LOBERG

GALLERY BOOKS

New York   London   Toronto   Sydney   New Delhi

G

Gallery Books
An Imprint of Simon & Schuster, Inc.
1230 Avenue of the Americas
New York, NY 10020

First Gallery Books hardcover edition December 2019

GALLERY BOOKS and colophon are registered trademarks of Simon & Schuster, Inc.

For information about special discounts for bulk purchases, please contact Simon & Schuster Special Sales at 1-866-506-1949 or business@simonandschuster.com.

The Simon & Schuster Speakers Bureau can bring authors to your live event. For more information or to book an event, contact the Simon & Schuster Speakers Bureau at 1-866-248-3049 or visit our website at www.simonspeakers.com.

Interior design by Davina Mock-Maniscalco

Manufactured in the United States of America

10   9   8   7   6   5   4   3   2   1

Library of Congress Cataloging-in-Publication Data is available.

ISBN 978-1-9821-1539-5
ISBN 978-1-9821-1541-8 (ebook)

To Durk Pearson and Sandy Shaw, whose early-1980s *Life Extension* books and newsletter inspired me to study this field.

And to Professors George Church and David Sinclair for encouraging me to turn my scientific notes on autophagy into a layman's book.

CONTENTS

CONTENTS

FOREWORD

I have spent my career steeped in the study of biology with a focus on the human genome—the genetic information, or DNA, we all carry in our cells that is the body's personal instruction manual. My mission is not only to learn how this marvelous, once mysterious code works and interacts with our environment, but to leverage its powers to enhance and extend people's youthful lives. My field of work has gone exponential in my lifetime, and especially in the past decade with the advent of economical DNA-sequencing techniques and gene-editing tools to hack a human body and change how we treat and prevent problems. Indeed, we are on the precipice of a whole new era of medicine, with studies coming out daily, sometimes hourly, that add fresh insights to our library of information on the human body and give us clues to outsmarting the aging process.

One of the most fascinating discoveries of late has been an intriguing process called autophagy. Although we in the scientific community have been studying this biological activity for decades, only in 2016 did the research finally culminate in a clear understanding about it and earn a Japanese cell biologist, Yoshinori Ohsumi, the Nobel Prize for his contributions. The word literally means "self-eating," but as you're about to read, it's not as horrifying as it sounds. Autophagy is simply the body's natural way of recycling and renewing its parts to avoid disease and dysfunction. It's a process that has been conserved in the genetic code of life for billions of years, so yes, it even predates us humans. We all would do well to keep our autophagy working properly, and I can't think of anyone more qualified to bring this important message to you than James Clement. In these pages you'll learn everything you need to know about autophagy and how to maximize your body's ability to repair its cells all the way down to your DNA.

I first met James in June 2009 when I read to him his genome interpretation (via Knome, the first direct-to-consumer whole genome sequencing company that I had just cofounded) at the Harvard Club in Boston. He later donated his genome to the Harvard Personal Genome Project where I am principal investigator. I started the PGP in 2005 with the goal of creating a public repository of human genomes to enable research into personal genomics and personalized medicine. We want to allow scientists to connect human genetic information with human trait information and environmental exposures. James was a very early adopter, being the twelfth person in the world to have his whole genome sequenced. I loved his drive to learn as much as he could about human biology and to push the limits of healthy life span. I knew he'd been a tax lawyer in his former life, and later a microbrewery owner and brewmaster, but I sensed he found his calling in biomedical research. And I've been known to support the scientific endeavors of innovative, bright people from diverse backgrounds and unexpected expertise.

In 2010, James came to me with a provocative question: Can we do gene editing on our own stem cells to iteratively make them better so that we could live longer? I told him this was a great idea but that we just didn't know which genes let people live longer, healthier lives. He came back a few months later with another idea that I couldn't resist participating in, and it revolved around another interesting question: What can we learn from the whole genomes of people who remain remarkably healthy into their first decade past 100? (We ended up focusing on people 106 years of age and older.) I became the first person to join the scientific advisory board for his Supercentenarian Research Study, later helping him recruit other advisers, mentoring him, and arranging for the gratis whole-genome sequencing of the last thirty-five samples by Veritas Genetics, a company I cofounded. Driven by his urgency to find answers, James then convinced me and his investors to make these genomes available for free to researchers around the world. To date he has collaborations with more than a dozen world-class institutions now combing this data set for valuable insights into healthy aging. The project has since spawned others for his nonprofit organization, which I'm also involved in, including studies that aim to radically extend healthy life spans, end human diseases, improve human cognition and well-being, and allow us to upgrade those biological features that are important to us.

I'm thrilled that James is on a mission to teach people how they can live long and well, even if they didn't win the genetic lottery. I've been encouraging James for years to write the book on autophagy for everyday folks and their physicians so they can discuss this knowledge. In this practical book, he shares insights into slowing aging, and possibly reversing it, by cycling back and forth between activating autophagy and mTOR, two very important cell processes you will learn about in this book. It's currently the best antiaging "switch" that we know of, and it already exists within you. Here is a riveting story about how to turn it on and know when to let it turn off. The strategies to do so are easy, accessible, and inexpensive.

James is one of the few researchers who shares my urgency with getting things done quickly and helping reduce human suffering while allowing people to live long past 100 in youthful health. A couple of years into the Supercentenarian Research Study, when he was approaching 60 years of age, he asked me if I thought he should take time off to get into a PhD program to fill in his knowledge base and help make him into a good scientist. I told him that he was already working on a project most graduate students would give their eyeteeth to be involved in, that he was reading as many scientific papers per day as anyone could, and most important, that a degree doesn't make a scientist—publishing peer-reviewed, scientific papers makes someone a scientist. He followed my advice and stuck with the study and has since branched off into other areas of antiaging research, coauthoring a growing number of scientific papers and fulfilling my prediction that he'd make a good scientist.

I think *The Switch* makes complex biology understandable and even engaging. You're about to learn a lot more about yourself and hopefully come to enjoy biology as much as James and I do. Autophagy is one of the body's health "codes," and the better we can harness its power, the better off we will be.

George M. Church
Professor of genetics, Harvard Medical School

INTRODUCTION

THE SWITCH

Life's tragedy is that we get old too soon and wise too late.
—Benjamin Franklin

A breakthrough in medical science quietly happened a few years ago that made the rounds in major scientific circles but somehow stayed a whisper in lay society. Let me ask you this: In your own grasp of the "secrets" of living a good, long life, what comes to mind? My bet is that you think of blood sugar balance, healthy weight, and physical fitness. Those are all appropriate goals to achieve, but they miss the main point—they are merely a means of sparking a prominent antiaging process: *autophagy.*[*] It's how the body removes and recycles dangerous, damaged organelles[†] and particles, as well as pathogens,[‡] from your cells, thus boosting your

---

[*]I prefer to pronounce the word "aw-*tof*-uh-jee."
[†]Any of a number of organized or specialized structures within a living cell.
[‡]Adversarial microbes that can cause disease.

1

immune system and greatly reducing your risk of developing cancer, heart disease, chronic inflammation, osteoarthritis, and neurological disorders from depression to dementia. Autophagy can be triggered when a certain complex, called mTOR, within cells is turned *down*. I refer to the mTOR complex as "the Switch."

Your body is made up of trillions of cells,* the majority of which consist of similar structures, carrying on similar activities. These structures are not just similar to other cells within you but exceedingly homologous to those of all of the other animals on our planet and largely comparable to bacteria, from which we evolved. Cells are perpetually carrying out a multitude of chemical reactions needed to keep the cell alive and healthy. This in turn keeps you alive. These chemical reactions share important relationships and are often connected through various pathways. The total reactions that take place inside of a cell are collectively called the cell's metabolism. The mTOR complex is one such pathway that takes place in nearly every cell. Virtually all health-extending and life span–extending interventions that we know of have their effects because of their actions to suppress this switch. Much of this book will be detailing how these various interventions, some of which you may have heard of and others of which you haven't, act on this pathway and ultimately regulate this important switch, periodically turning on autophagy in the process.

Think of this switch like a dimmer for your lights: turning it toward one end to increase light and the other direction to decrease

---

*The actual number of cells in the average human body is still debated among scientists. Although it remains a mystery, most would agree that the number is between 30 and 40 trillion, but that doesn't include the bacteria that are present in and on our bodies.

it. Although we evolved to have this biological switch move back and forth continuously between growth (mTOR) and repair (autophagy; and sometimes repair for prolonged periods), the lifestyles of modern humans keep it turned toward growth constantly and seldom or never in the repair direction. And when it's in the growth stage, these cellular garbage trucks come to a halt and our ability to clear out the biological debris—misfolded proteins, pathogens, and dysfunctional organelles—falters. The word *autophagy* literally means "self-eating" in Greek and refers to the body's powerful, self-cleaning switch inside most cells. Information about this vital internal degradation system has been documented for decades, but only in the past few years have we figured out how and why it functions. In 2016, understanding autophagy's mechanisms in the body earned the Japanese cell biologist Dr. Yoshinori Ohsumi of the Tokyo Institute of Technology a Nobel Prize in Physiology or Medicine. His work unraveled the mechanism of autophagy and has led to a new paradigm in medicine, one that is being hailed as *the* discovery of the twenty-first century.

THE TWENTY-FIRST-CENTURY PARADOX

If you are over the age of twenty-five, I have some unfortunate news for you: you are technically "aging" now. That's not to say you haven't been aging since the day you were born. But certain biological events switched gears two and a half decades after your birth that physically put you onto the inevitable descending slope of your life's arc. Your cellular processes changed, your growth hormones shifted levels (after all, you're not getting any taller or moving up in shoe sizes anymore), your metabolism ticked down a notch, your brain neared its final structural formation, and your muscle and bone mass peaked. By the time you see that first wrinkle, lack a healthy glow because you stayed up late last night, feel ten pounds heavier than in your high school days, or experience a symptom such as unexplained low energy and insomnia, these outward cues have long been in development somewhere deep inside. They don't happen overnight, even though it may seem that way.

We live in exciting times for personal health, thanks to the speed at which analytical and diagnostic technologies are adding to scientific advancements in knowledge about the human body. The crude and often expensive chemical, molecular, and optical instruments used in the twentieth century have given way to highly precise, affordable tools in the twenty-first. I have a laboratory full of such equipment, unheard of in private labs just a few decades ago. Papers of well-designed studies in the field of biology and medicine are being published at an exponential rate. And we are rapidly entering a new age of controlling our disease risk and life span. As a result, scientists' understanding of the activities inside our cells has been skyrocketing. For the most part, however, this important new information, which should impact many of our lifestyle and health care decisions, is unknown to the government officials making health care recommendations and the physicians who care for us. We need this knowledge in order to inform the choices we make that relate to wellness. Although we no longer worry about dying from communicable or infectious diseases as we did in 1900, we increasingly suffer from overconsumption of the wrong sorts of foods and reduced levels of healthy activities. But these age-related illnesses are largely preventable

4

through changes in our diet and lifestyle and the use of revolutionary drugs and certain supplements.

In 2019, one of the most prestigious medical journals, *The Lancet*, published an alarming study stating that fully 1 in 5 deaths globally are now the result of unhealthy diets alone.[1] This is not due primarily to lack of access to good, nutritious food; people are eating too much sugar, salt, and meat, which contribute to heart disease, cancer, diabetes, and dementia—the major maladies of our twenty-first-century civilization. That means 11 million people are prematurely wiped off the planet each year because they do not consume the right foods. That's more deaths from poor dietary choices than from tobacco smoking or high blood pressure. The study even managed to take into consideration age, gender, country of residence, and socioeconomic status. People are affected by bad eating habits *despite* these factors, meaning that diet is the leading cause of chronic disease in the world today—a shameful fact given that we do not have to forage for food anymore.

That study came on the heels of another led by the University of North Carolina at Chapel Hill's Gillings School of Global Public Health that identified the percentage of Americans who are metabolically healthy.[2] Being metabolically healthy is defined as having ideal levels of five parameters without the aid of drugs: blood glucose, triglycerides (blood fats), high-density lipoprotein (HDL, or "good") cholesterol, blood pressure, and waist circumference. The study mined data from the National Health and Nutrition Examination Survey that included 8,721 people in the United States between 2009 and 2016. The goal was to determine how many adults are at low versus high risk for chronic disease.

The results, based on a sophisticated calculation, was that only 12.2 percent of Americans, or 1 in 8, are in a state of optimal metabolic health—yet another shameful fact given that these aspects are well within our control.

And it's not just the wrong foods that are killing us; it's portion sizes. Foods today are often intentionally engineered for overconsumption. We've become overfed and undernourished. It's a modern paradox: we can enjoy a much healthier diet than ever before thanks to easy access to a panoply of nutritious natural foods coupled with advanced farming and distribution practices that allow us to buy, for example, fresh fruits and vegetables year-round. But at the same time, our diets are becoming less healthy and dangerously high in calories. It pains me to watch someone order a plateful of fluffy buttermilk pancakes doused with lots of syrup (made with corn syrup) and a side of bacon, followed by an order of cheese pizza. Yes, I have witnessed this, and all I see is diabetes on a plate with heart disease for dessert. We deserve better.

It doesn't help that there is also enormous confusion on the subject of diet, causing tremendous anxiety among people who are trying to do better for their waistlines and health. Look no further than the low-carb versus low-fat or vegan versus carnivore movements to see the debates. We are bombarded by mixed messages in the media as well as by dubious claims made by food manufacturers. I find it mind-boggling how polarizing and political the topic of nutrition has become. Food should be a source of joy and sustenance, not fear and disease. Too rarely do we think about the connection between what we eat and our risk of developing certain ailments. We know that smoking causes lung cancer, but how does consuming too many sodas, bagels, or cheeseburgers increase our chances of developing Alzheimer's disease, heart disease, or colon cancer? The links are not so obvious.

The modern food-processing industry and misleading marketing have contributed to making Americans progressively sicker. But I have good news for you: we can change.

A SELF-PROFESSED CITIZEN SCIENTIST

I grew up in the 1960s and '70s, a typical midwestern science nerd (especially anything having to do with space or brain science). In college I majored in political science and psychology (emphasis on neurophysiology), and in my sophomore year I worked on a project with a neurophysiologist that earned me a coauthorship of a paper published in the journal *Science*. After graduating, I worked for a year for the Missouri senate president pro tem and then went to law school. In my final year at the University of California Hastings College of the Law in San Francisco, I read and was deeply inspired by Durk Pearson and Sandy Shaw's *Life Extension: A Scientific Practical Approach*. My wife, who was also a law student at the time, talked me out of shifting careers to become a molecular biologist. But that ambition burned in me for the next two decades. After years of practicing law and then starting and running various businesses (including an iconic brewpub near the Cornell University campus in Ithaca, New York), I eventually returned to that dream.

In the early 2000s, I got involved in the nascent life extension movement. I volunteered for a few longevity-oriented organizations and later ran the World Transhumanist Association, an organization dedicated to overcoming our biological limitations with the aid of technology. With my good friend Dan Stoicescu, I co-founded *h+ Magazine*, which we ran for the next few years, with R. U. Sirius as our editor. (Dr. Stoicescu has a doctorate in medicinal chemistry and was the second person in the world to buy the full sequence of his own genetic code and pay the hefty price tag at the time of $350,000.) With Dan's encouragement and support, I spent most of 2008 and 2009 attending biotech and medical conferences, visiting the labs of people working on stem cell research, cloning, and gene therapy, and reading scientific papers in diverse areas related to maintaining health and longevity. I was hooked.

In November 2009, I attended the first-ever Executive Program at Singularity University, a futurist-oriented Silicon Valley–based business incubator set up by Peter Diamandis and Ray Kurzweil to solve the world's problems through the use of what's called exponential technology. Exponential technologies are those that are accelerating rapidly and shaping major industries and all aspects of our lives. They include technologies such as artificial intelligence (AI), augmented and virtual reality, big data science and medicine, robotics, and autonomous vehicles. Diamandis and Kurzweil encouraged their students to think in terms of helping $10^{9\text{th}}$ (a billion) people, on any project they chose. I decided then and there that I wanted to focus all my future efforts on increasing healthy life span for everyone.

In early 2010, I set up the Supercentenarian Research Study to find out how individuals who lived past 105 years of age had avoided life-threatening diseases such as cancer, heart disease, and neurodegenerative disorders. I was able to get the support of top scientists, including George Church of Harvard Medical School and João Pedro de Magalhães of the University of Liverpool, who continue to serve as scientific advisers to my nonprofit medical research organization. During the next several years, a colleague and I traveled around North America and Europe collecting more than sixty blood samples from individuals 106 years of age and older.

Starting in December 2009, I began reading five to ten scientific papers a day related to the biology of aging. By June 2019, I had read more than eighteen thousand such papers. In 2013, I decided to take a deep dive into the science of dietary restriction (caloric and protein), fasting (intermittent and prolonged), and the ketogenic (very-low-carbohydrate) diet, with which I had recently started self-experimenting. What I wanted to know was the following: What causes the beneficial effects of these diets? And do these three practices improve health and life span via similar or different mechanisms?

This book attempts to answer these questions, because five hundred papers into this quest, I realized that the intracellular complex called mTOR and the process that's initiated whenever it's turned down—autophagy—might be the secret of a longer, healthier life. As I came to find out, changing the direction of this metabolic switch is the primary reason that calorie restriction, intermittent fasting, and very-low-carb diets can be so beneficial to extending life. I read another five hundred papers to try to poke holes in that hypothesis, and in December 2013 I presented my findings to my mentor, Dr. George Church, professor of genetics at Harvard Medical School, and Dr. David Sinclair, a friend and another famous professor at that school. They both agreed that I was onto something and encouraged me to follow my research as far as I could. David is the one who encouraged me to write this book to share my knowledge with other scientists, medical professionals, and the public. Meanwhile, the literature on mTOR and autophagy was exploding, and I soon found myself steeped in studies while continuing to follow the trail of radical life extension. (As an aside: I am Harvard Personal Genome Project participant number 145, and my PGP ID is hu82E689. If you're interested, you can download my full genome, mutations, and health data at https://my.pgp-hms.org/profile/hu82E689. Bragging rights: I was the twelfth person in the world to have his or her whole genome sequenced, in early 2010.)

I currently run a 501(c)(3) nonprofit medical research organization called Betterhumans (https://betterhumans.org), focused on extending healthy human life span and reducing disease risk. I also serve as the principal investigator of several Institutional Review Board–approved human clinical trials and oversee my own laboratory, which engages in a broad range of antiaging experiments and basic research. Since devoting my life to studying life extension, the number of my projects has skyrocketed through collaborations with some of the world's most respected scientists in high-profile labs at Harvard, Yale, Scripps Research Institute, UCLA, the University of New South Wales, Mount Sinai Hospital, Princeton, and the University of Texas Southwestern Medical Center.

I believe current advancements in medical science will bring about revolutionary life extension (living healthy well beyond 100 years), and I want to help it arrive quickly enough so that my parents (in their late 80s), my elderly friends, and even the wonderful and vibrant centenarians and supercentenarians I've met will have the chance to live much longer, truly healthy (as healthy as they were in their 30s) life spans. I have no doubt that this will change society, and I'm not at all convinced—as some are—that society's future will be a dystopian, Malthusian one.

I also want to reach younger generations. We now know that people in their 30s and 40s could be in the early stages of developing dementia, cancer, and heart disease, though it could take years, and in some cases decades, for them or their doctors to realize this. With proper lifestyle choices, individuals in their 50s can live well into their 70s, 80s, and longer feeling as though they are still only at the halfway century mark. Previously, it was thought that only about 65 to 75 percent of longevity was attributable to lifestyle, with the rest being genetic. Newer research blows this percentage up to more than 90 percent.[3] For most people (who aren't lucky enough to inherit supercentenarian genes), that's a very good thing, because it means that healthy longevity is within our control, if we can muster the desire and self-discipline to attain it.

Fewer than 50 percent of people who live in the United States today make it to the average age at death of 82, and two-thirds of those will die of cancer or heart disease, with many of the "lucky half" who make it past 82 succumbing to sarcopenia (loss of muscle tissue), osteoporosis (loss of bone density), hypertension, dementia, Parkinson's disease, or Alzheimer's disease. It doesn't have to be this way. Cancer, heart disease, and Alzheimer's are still rare in many "primitive" parts of the world, including small regions of even modernized countries. In these "longevity oases," as many as three times the number of people reach the age of 100 and beyond, retaining their memories and good health much longer than we do. To say I'm on a mission to rectify this discrepancy and bring back good health and longevity to people suffering from the "diseases of civilization" is an understatement.

Multiple clinical trials are in motion today throughout the world based on the heart of this book's theme: how to lengthen your life without having the genes of a supercentenarian by leveraging the power of autophagy, a process that should be taking place in your body on a daily basis but has probably been turned off—lying dormant—for years. I'll show you how to turn it back on.

IN THIS BOOK

I'm going to explain how a Canadian research expedition from McGill University to the remote Easter Island in the 1970s led to the initial clues to this important cellular switch. I'll show how scientific research on yeast, worms, and fruit flies has revealed that autophagy is crucial to the health and longevity benefits derived from calorie restriction, intermittent fasting, and exercise. You'll learn how genetically modified mice strains and humans with rare mutant genes are protected from cancer, heart disease, diabetes, and neurological diseases, because of this same self-cleaning switch. I'll also explain why the science of nutrition has not yet caught up with these valuable data and why money and politics are aligned to continue recommending diets that are not consistent with keeping you healthy. (Even the popular Paleolithic or "paleo"* and vegan

---

*The Paleolithic diet, or the diet that mimics how humans ate during that epoch in our evolution—from 2.6 million years ago to the dawn of agriculture about 12,000 years ago—is often referred to simply as the "paleo" diet in our culture today. Going forward, I am going to call it the paleo diet in the book.

diets are flawed for reasons I will explain.) Each chapter takes you on what I hope to be a riveting tour of an important piece of this biological phenomenon.

At the end of the book, I'll give you a general framework to follow that puts all the ideas into actionable form. There will be times when you will not want autophagy running high in your body, and I'll explain why. All of the strategies are simply meant to mimic the natural processes that animals (including humans) undergo when living in the natural environment. Our modern farming and food preservation technologies and conveniences have paradoxically led to accelerated aging due to the availability of unlimited quantities of very quickly digestible foods, especially sugar (including high-fructose corn syrup), simple carbohydrates, grain-fed meats (full of the wrong kinds of fats), and lots of dairy products (loaded with proteins that keep the Switch turned in the growth direction). There is also something to be said for the terrible lack of fiber in our diets that affects the health of our digestive system and microbial comrades collectively called the microbiome. Your gut plays an enormous, underappreciated role in your metabolism and risk of developing disease. The information in this book is meant to help reverse this hastening of aging and put us back onto a more natural path of consumption and exercise that keeps the Switch (mTOR and autophagy) in balance and prevents the age-related diseases that were rare centuries ago but are widespread now.

Although there is much to be learned in this emerging field, especially regarding the stimulation and optimization of this cellular activity, the good news is that you can take advantage of what we've already discovered starting today. These recommendations will include what to do and not to do with regard to your nutrition, medications, vitamins and supplements, and general lifestyle choices. Some of the recommendations will be downright surprising. Who knew that a smidgen of certain toxins can be good for you and that there's one particular nut that deserves a halo? Who knew that popular versions of the paleo or hunter-gatherer diet, which are all the rage today, could be putting you at risk of having high blood sugar, weight gain, bone decline, kidney challenges, and cancerous growths?

I believe, as do many researchers in this field, that the mechanism that controls this switch is one of the most important discoveries in modern medicine. The application of this knowledge in our daily habits can "square the mortality curve"* by helping individuals age without experiencing the debilitating and costly effects of lifestyle-related diseases. I hope that shining a spotlight on this scarcely known process will also encourage doctors to educate their patients and incorporate this information into their advice and treatment protocols. And I hope that by bringing greater awareness to this narrow field, more scientists will study how this biological machinery is involved in and affected by their own research experiments as well as spur additional private and government funding for further research.

---

*"Squaring the mortality curve" means that your morbidity risk remains low as you grow old, and rather than your becoming increasingly frailer as you age, your good health lasts right up until a short time before your death. This is how many supercentenarians experience death.

CHAPTER 1

EASTER ISLAND AND
TRANSPLANT PATIENTS

The first time the concept of the Switch entered my mind, I was reading a paper by Professor Stephen Spindler of the University of California, Riverside, on how calorie restriction (CR) prevented cancer in mice.[1] It was probably the five hundredth paper I'd devoured in 2013 about the subjects of CR, fasting, ketogenesis, and longevity, as I'd become a little obsessed with figuring out how I could help my parents live past 100 without suffering from our modern scourges: diabetes, heart disease, and dementia. I came across the usual tips: avoid refined, processed foods, especially those filled with sugar, fat, and salt; stay active; sleep well; don't smoke; and don't drink too much alcohol. But I also encountered a lot of material buried in the scientific literature that I'd never heard about and that was both indisputable and compelling. Believe it or not, there's solid evidence that you'll want to favor certain nuts over others, that consuming too much protein can be damaging (and some specific animal-based proteins are much worse than others), that eating multiple small meals throughout the day is not ideal, that certain vitamins, such as vitamin E, can *increase* your risk of developing cancer, and that smoking a cigar once in a blue moon might actually help you live longer!

Facing data like that only made me want to dig deeper and further understand the workings of the body and its chances of remaining young from a cellular standpoint. And then one day, it finally hit me: all of the personal research I'd conducted and all the copious pages I'd read were pointing squarely to the Switch, a single mechanism in the body that turns up one process while it turns down the other and vice versa. Technically, the Switch is a protein complex called mTOR, short for **m**echanistic (formerly known as **m**ammalian) **T**arget **O**f **R**apamycin. As I briefly mentioned in the introduction, mTOR is the switch that nearly every cell (except blood cells) has, and it either activates your cell's self-cleaning mode (autophagy), ridding the body of toxic materials and fomenting cancers as well as burning fat, or allows the body to produce more proteins, store as much energy (glucose and fat) as possible, and build more cells. (Sometimes you do want to produce more proteins, store more fat, and build more cells—see chapter 9—but not to the perpetual exclusion of cellular repair and self-cleaning.) These anabolic processes, when taken to an extreme level, which our modern lifestyle practices do, can trigger illness.

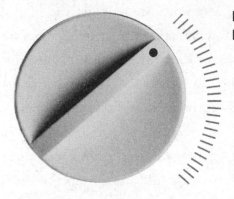

House Cleaning and Fat Burning (Autophagy)

Fat Storage and Muscle Building (mTOR)

The *R* in mTOR represents, as previously stated, *rapamycin*, a compound that's actually produced by a bacterium. To gain a full understanding of mTOR and put this concept of a cellular switch into greater perspective, let's take a brief journey back in time. The start of this detective story begins with a powerful invention: the electron microscope.

SEEING THE UNSEEABLE

The development of the electron microscope in the early part of the twentieth century helped trigger many paradigm shifts in medicine. It was possible largely due to the advent of electromagnetic lenses. Using magnetic lenses to focus and direct beams of electrons, whose wavelengths are 1/100,000th those of light waves, these microscopes can achieve magnification up to 10 million times. They allow us to see things that are invisible to normal microscopes, such as bacteria, viruses, and tiny cellular parts. In 1955, Christian de Duve, a scientist at the Catholic University of Louvain in Belgium, and Alex Novikoff, a scientist from the University of Vermont College of Medicine, used an electron microscope to detect, for the first time, membrane-like barriers within cells that sequester compounds and digest them. Duve named this organelle a lysosome, meaning "to loosen body," to describe its digestive properties, and in 1974 won a Nobel Prize in Physiology or Medicine for this discovery.

In 1961, Dr. Keith Porter, a pioneer in electron microscopy at the Rockefeller Institute in New York, and his postdoctoral student Thomas Ashford used an electron microscope to examine rat liver cells that were suffused with glucagon, a hormone made by the pancreas that, among other things, causes glucose to be produced by the liver and released into the bloodstream. Porter and Ashford are credited with being the first scientists to observe autophagy, though it would take decades longer to understand it.

A TALE OF TWO HORMONES

The hormone glucagon is produced by the alpha cells in the islets of Langerhans in the pancreas.

Glucagon secretion is stimulated by the ingestion of protein, by a low blood glucose concentration (hypoglycemia), and by exercise. It is inhibited by the ingestion of carbohydrates.

Insulin is produced by the beta cells in the islets of Langerhans in response to food, especially carbohydrates. Its role is to lower glucose levels in the bloodstream and promote the storage of glucose in fat, muscle, liver, and other body tissues.

Glucagon is the yin to insulin's yang. It strongly opposes the action of insulin, raising the concentration of glucose in the bloodstream by promoting the breakdown of glycogen (the form in which glucose is stored in liver, muscle, and fat cells) and by stimulating the production of glucose from amino acids and glycerol in the liver, a process called gluconeogenesis. By increasing the concentration of glucose in the bloodstream, glucagon serves the main role in maintaining blood glucose concentrations during fasting and exercise.

Once in the bloodstream in sufficient quantities, insulin, another hormone made by the pancreas, alerts cells to the presence of glucose in the bloodstream, so that insulin-dependent cells can bring the glucose into themselves to burn as fuel. This takes place in the cells' mitochondria. (As I'll describe later, the mitochondria are important intracellular organelles that produce energy.) Insulin and glucagon are closely tied together but generally work as two ends of a spectrum—in which the amount of glucose in the bloodstream is the deciding factor as to which is turned on: too low, and glucagon is released in order to cause the production of more glucose; when a high enough level of glucose in the bloodstream is attained, insulin is released. With the aid of an electron microscope, Ashford and Porter were able to observe certain membranes within cells that were in various stages of being degraded, or broken down. They also noted that it had recently been documented in medical literature that glucagon breaks down proteins

via this same process. The next year, after reading that German scientists had observed small, specialized membrane-degrading structures within cells called organelles when cells were injured or starved, Duve coined the term "autophagy" to describe the process of creating membranes, sequestering compounds, and digesting the targeted compounds.

It wasn't until a decade later that one of the key cellular mechanisms involved in turning autophagy off, mTOR, would be elucidated through another discovery, this one serendipitously found in the soil of a remote island that's just fourteen miles long and seven miles wide.

THE DISCOVERY OF THE SWITCH

Easter Island is a small volcanic island in the southeastern Pacific originally settled by Polynesians in the first millennium CE and called Rapa Nui by the natives (meaning "Navel of the World"). It's more than 2,000 miles off the coast of South America and 1,100 miles from its nearest Polynesian neighbor, Pitcairn Island, where mutineers from the famous Royal Navy ship HMS *Bounty* hid in the nineteenth century. At one time the original inhabitants numbered over 15,000, but when the Dutch explorer Jacob Roggeveen discovered it on Easter Sunday 1722, there were only a few thousand Polynesians left. To commemorate the date, he named it Easter Island. Today it's a World Heritage Site owned by Chile, famous for its archaeological ruins, including nearly nine hundred monumental statues called *moai*, created by inhabitants during the thirteenth to sixteenth centuries.

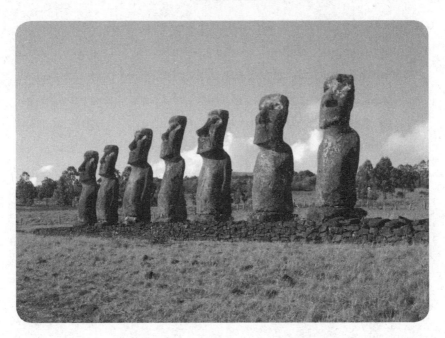

In 1972, Canadian researchers from McGill University took soil samples on Easter Island and discovered *Streptomyces hygroscopicus*, a bacterial species that secretes a compound to stop the growth of competitive fungi and to absorb as many nutrients as possible for itself. The researchers named this compound rapamycin in honor of the island's native name. Rapamycin was shown to act similar to an antibiotic, with powerful antibacterial, antifungal, and immunosuppressive effects. Dr. Suren Sehgal at Ayerst Research Laboratories in Montreal, where rapamycin was isolated later that year, observed that the compound possessed tumor-suppressing attributes; he sent a sample to the US National Cancer Institute (NCI).[2] Rapamycin did so well at inhibiting numerous cancer cell lines that the NCI advanced it as a priority drug for development.

In the early 1980s, labs began studying rapamycin, and over the next decade a stream of scientific papers came out reporting its inhibitory effect on cell growth in yeast, fruit flies, round-worms, fungi, plants, and, most important for us, mammals. (It wasn't until 1994 that scientists finally discovered the mammalian version of TOR thanks to the work of David Sabatini and his colleagues at Johns Hopkins University School of Medicine and the Memorial Sloan Kettering Cancer Center in New York.)[3] In all of those organisms, the inhibitory mechanism involves binding to the target proteins, collectively named "target of rapamycin" (TOR). Put simply, rapamycin binds to TOR as a key fits into a lock, and in doing so, TOR activity is lowered. (Note: For purposes of this discussion going forward, I will use the more precise term "mTOR," with "m" standing for "mechanistic" because that is how it's referred to in the literature and we are talking primarily about how TOR operates in humans.)

The discovery of rapamycin, which led to the discovery of mTOR, allowed scientists to begin mapping out the biological pathways leading to the activation or, conversely, inhibition of mTOR and the resulting effects. One such observation was that when mTOR was activated, autophagy was suppressed, and when mTOR was silenced, autophagy was enhanced. This controls, in some sense, whether the cell is in an *anabolic* (growth) phase or in a *catabolic* (housecleaning) phase. It helps to think of mTOR functions as the central hub of the cell signaling system, the command and control center of the cell. There's a reason why it's been conserved through 2 billion years of evolution: a master regulator of cell growth and metabolism, it's one of the secrets of how cell metabolism—life—is orchestrated within the cell. And it is the essence of the Switch.

Today rapamycin is used in organ transplant patients to prevent rejection and has become one of the hottest antiaging and anticancer drugs under investigation. Because it has extended the life span of every living thing tested in the laboratory, it's also being researched for its ability to reduce the risk of developing diabetes, heart disease, neurodegenerative ailments, immune system decline, and accelerated aging in general. I myself am currently conducting a series of clinical trials to see whether long-term intermittent (once-per-week) use of rapamycin by elderly people will protect them from age-related disease. Numerous other studies are being conducted around the world to examine the drug's many positive effects on human biology. Let's review a few of the key findings, especially with regard to life extension.

RAPAMYCIN AND AGING

The discovery of rapamycin's power over cellular processes started with an enigma. In the 1990s, Zelton Dave Sharp, a pharmacologist at the Sam and Ann Barshop Institute for Longevity and Aging Studies at the University of Texas Health Science Center at San Antonio, was studying mice that had a peculiar condition called pituitary dwarfism. These mice do not make enough growth hormone for normal development due to a defect in their pituitary gland.[4] Though they might have been lacking in size, the dwarf mice made up for that shortcoming with impressive longevity, living longer than normal mice. Was there a connection? How could a genetic error that caused an animal to be abnormally small also abnormally lengthen life?

Flash forward to 1996, when Michael Hall, a molecular biologist at the Biozentrum at the University of Basel in Switzerland, led a team of scientists who found a new biological pathway in yeast that was controlled by the protein targets of rapamycin.[5] They revealed that when they used rapamycin to block these proteins in yeast, it produced the same effect as if the yeast had been starved. The yeast cells lived longer than normal cells, and they were smaller. (Dr. Hall won an Albert Lasker Basic Medical Research Award in 2017 for his work.) Hall's finding stirred Sharp's scientifically minded imagination. He wondered if mTOR was a "nutrient response system," whereby there was a relationship between diet restriction and growth factor restriction (growth factors are the necessary substances to stimulate many aspects of cellular function including proliferation, differentiation, and survival). He then predicted that the mice would live a long time if they ingested rapamycin. That was where the contradiction came in: How could a drug used for decades to dampen the immune system simultaneously extend life?

But Sharp was onto something, and he didn't abandon his quest, ultimately playing a role in establishing the data to demonstrate this profound conundrum. In the early 2000s, studies demonstrated that rapamycin can make worms and fruit flies live longer.[6] Research not just by Sharp but by others also indicated that mTOR signaling was downregulated in dwarf mice. "Signaling" simply means the chain of effects, or communication processes, between molecules or cells; "downregulated" essentially means that the signaling is hushed. What followed was a collaboration among Sharp, Randy Strong, the principal investigator for the National Institute on Aging's Interventions Testing Program, and David Harrison, a scientist at the Jackson Laboratory in Bar Harbor, Maine. Their work resulted in a noteworthy mouse study that singled out rapamycin as a potential substance to extend life span in mammals, the first of its kind. The study was published in the prestigious journal *Nature* in 2009 and included about a dozen other researchers from various institutions across the United States.[7]

The design and scope of that study made the results all the more compelling. While one group of researchers bred the mice to be used in the study, another worked on preparing the rapamycin for the experiment. Each lab bred its own mice from an original stock supplied by the Jackson Lab, which helped rule out the possibility that the drug might work for one group of mice but not others. Originally, the therapy was to begin when the mice were about 4 months old (youthful adults), but the amount of rapamycin required to sustain the levels needed in the blood of the mice turned out to be prohibitively expensive, since most of the drug was destroyed in the stomach before it could reach the intestines, where it could be absorbed. The researchers therefore set out to find a way to reduce the cost by making it survive stomach acids. By the time the consortium of researchers solved the problem by microencapsulating the rapamycin in a polymer coating that disintegrated only in the intestine of the mice, the mice were much older. Rather than breed a whole new group of mice for the experiments, they decided to go ahead and see what happened when they gave the rapamycin to old-aged (20-month-old) mice—the equivalent of a human nearing seventy.

Supplementing the mice with rapamycin resulted in extending the life span of male mice by 9 percent and female mice by 14 percent. The experiment was the first time that a drug was shown to enhance longevity in a mammal. Previously, life span in mice had been increased only by calorie restriction or genetic manipulation.

Fearing that rapamycin might interfere with the production of mitochondrial DNA or protein levels, Harrison was part of a team that later tested the drug on mice and examined the mitochondria in their skeletal muscles.[8] They found no consistent changes in those levels and also documented that treated mice had treadmill endurance equal to that of the controls—a good indication that their mitochondria were operating as well as those of nontreated mice.

In 2012, Dr. Harrison and the group of researchers from the 2009 study, this time including Dr. J. Erby Wilkinson, a pathologist from the University of Michigan Animal Care & Use Program, fed enteric-coated rapamycin to 9-month-old mice until they were 22 months old (before any control mice or rapamycin-fed mice in the previous study had died), and compared them to young (4-month-old) mice to see how they had aged.[9] Their results showed that rapamycin-treated mice were delayed in the development of many forms of age-related diseases, including degenerative changes in the liver, heart, and joints. In their conclusions, the researchers went so far as to suggest that the rapamycin had anti-cancer effects as well. They wrote, "Rapamycin may well both slow multiple aspects of aging and also have a direct anti-tumor effect." They also suggested that the anticancer effects could have merely been an automatic result of the delayed aging itself rather than being a direct effect.

As is said in biomedical research, game-changing results are useful and informative only when they can be repeated by other scientists. In 2009, an independent group led by Chong Chen at the University of Michigan's Division of Immunotherapy also showed increased life span in aged mice given rapamycin.[10] A breed of mice different from those used in the NIA study were treated with rapamycin every other day for six weeks starting at age 22 months. Over the next thirty weeks, the mice had a significantly increased survival rate compared with placebo-injected controls. This treatment protocol was also shown to boost the function of certain stem cells in the aged mice and enhance responses to the influenza vaccine. Such effects protected the aged mice from a potentially lethal infection.

When the NIA-led group repeated their experiment, this time using a dose of rapamycin that was three times higher than the previous experiment, they managed to increase the average life span of male mice by a jaw-dropping 23 percent and female mice by 26 percent.[11] That's pretty significant.

Researchers have now further explored the study of rapamycin's life span–extending benefits to other animal species. An ongoing collaboration between the University of Washington's Healthy Aging and Longevity Research Institute and Texas A&M University College of Veterinary Medicine, for example, is studying the effects of rapamycin in dogs.[12] It's not known yet if the drug will extend the healthy life span, or health span, of the animals, but scientists have already documented interesting findings, such as measurable improvements in cardiac function after ten weeks on the drug. Texas A&M's Kate Creevy, the chief medical officer for the Dog Aging Project,[13] hopes to move the drug toward approval for use as a veterinary medicine, following appropriate clinical trials, in order to continue their investigations. But studies like this will bring to light how the drug can help humans, too. Dogs can be much better proxies than other laboratory animals because they are more genetically diverse. I should also give credit to Mikhail Blagosklonny, a scientist now at Roswell Park

Comprehensive Cancer Center in Buffalo, New York, who focuses on life extension and cancer prevention. He contributed greatly to establishing the importance of rapamycin and mTOR in the scientific literature. His 2006 paper was among the first to state that aging is a disease process caused by overactive mTOR.[14]

Still missing from all this groundbreaking research, however, is a behind-the-scenes biological understanding of how rapamycin extends life span. What does it actually do to prolong life? How does it function? Part of the problem comes from the fact that the pathway it acts upon is involved in multiple biochemical processes. Its target, mTOR, is a large protein complex located in the cytoplasm of the cell, right next to the nucleus. It operates in close communication with the nucleus of the cell, sensing what is happening within the cell and then signaling the nucleus how to respond. mTOR is used in a myriad of activities throughout the body—in the nervous system, the muscles, and all of the organs—so teasing out the exact mechanisms of its effects in the aging process is an enormous challenge. No doubt future research will suss this out.

Although human clinical trials for healthy longevity are difficult to fund, studies on the various health benefits of rapamycin for humans (primarily reducing various disease risks) are gaining traction. There's just too much at stake here to ignore. At this writing, more than 1,300 clinical trials are taking place using rapamycin for everything from Crohn's disease and cancer to Alzheimer's disease. What started as a drug chiefly for transplant patients is showing promise to help the rest of us. Perhaps we can use it to "transplant" forces inside us that would otherwise shorten our lives so that we can live both longer and better.

Now, I may have painted a picture of rapamycin that makes it sound like the fountain of youth. Should we all be taking this drug to prolong our lives? Not necessarily. But what we do want is to control its power in the body: autophagy.

If rapamycin can reduce the risk of degenerative diseases and promote health via autophagy, what exactly is autophagy and how does it work?

CHAPTER 2

GARBAGE TRUCKS AND RECYCLING PLANTS

s we all know, obesity has become a major problem throughout much of the world, especially in first-world countries where the Western diet prevails. Rates of obesity have nearly tripled since 1975 and know no boundaries—obesity is pandemic in all industrialized nations, across all age groups, and in both urban and rural areas. In fact, contrary to popular wisdom, which says that urbanization has driven our obesity epidemic in the past several decades, new large-scale research proves otherwise. Rural residents are now gaining weight at a faster rate than city slickers, becoming the main drivers of this modern plague. And despite trillions of dollars having been spent on research and drug development, the risk of developing cancer, heart disease, and Alzheimer's disease has continued to increase and appears to be linked to dangerous excess weight (Alzheimer's is sometimes referred to medically as type 3 diabetes).

Everything I'd been reading told me that these ailments were also related to aging itself. Very few people get these diseases when they're young. Yet the more I learned, the more I realized the complexity of the problem. Two things, however, kept playing in the back of my mind. The first was that researchers discovered nearly eighty years ago that both calorie restriction (CR) and intermittent fasting (IF) greatly extended the lives of test animals, often by reducing their vulnerability to cancer and heart disease. A ketogenic (very-low-carbohydrate) diet, widely used for the treatment of neurological diseases, showed somewhat similar anticancer and anti–heart disease benefits, although it has been investigated much less than CR or IF. The second was that two uncommon gene variations had already been discovered in supercentenarians that appeared to protect them from diseases. Those genes (FOXO3 and IGF-1) were impacted by those diets and linked to their effects on blood sugar and insulin.

I then dug deeper into the scientific data, learning as much as I could about calorie restriction, intermittent fasting, and ketogenic diets. The question that I was curious about, and which I mentioned earlier, was whether the diets worked by the same mechanism or differently. After three months of reading through more than five hundred scientific papers, it finally dawned on me that all of the papers I'd been reading about life-extending, disease-preventing genes, therapies, drugs, vitamins/supplements, lifestyles, and so on had one thing in common: they turned down the mTOR cellular mechanism and thereby turned up the autophagy process. I spent another three months reading six hundred more papers focused on mTOR and autophagy, and confirmed my suspicion. The primary, but not exclusive, means of turning on autophagy was by blocking the effect that insulin and the related insulin-like growth factor 1 (also known as IGF-1) had on keeping mTOR activated and the cell stuck in "production" mode.

In this chapter we'll take a closer look at the process of autophagy—the natural, expertly controlled, destructive mechanism of the cell that disassembles unnecessary or dysfunctional components, including faulty organelles, misfolded proteins, and pathogens. As I've already defined, it's the process by which your body continually detoxifies, repairs, and ultimately regenerates itself. Some of the substances that result from the degradation are reused to produce new proteins, some of which may go into making new organelles, such as mitochondria. Researchers increasingly credit autophagy with playing a role in many biological processes from the moment of conception. It affects development, aging, cellular renewal, and immunity. Its dysfunction appears to be a guilty party in conditions as diverse as inflammatory diseases, cancer, and neurodegeneration, including ailments such as Parkinson's and Alzheimer's. Although the term "autophagy" was coined more than half a century ago by Christian de Duve to describe the process that cells use to break down and recycle their components, not until recently did scientists unravel all the moving parts to this process. It's really no wonder that the field of autophagy is growing immensely to include scientists of "all flavors," as the cancer biologist Kay Macleod of the Ben May Department for Cancer Research at the University of Chicago phrases it.[1] Everyone wants to get into the game.

Though autophagy is a complex process that serves a lot of diverse roles in the body, it helps to think of it simply as our innate recycling machinery—a process of intracellular housekeeping. Autophagy makes us more physiologically efficient by getting rid of defective parts, promoting healthy metabolism, stopping cancerous growths, and preventing metabolic disorders such as obesity and diabetes—which means that by boosting your body's autophagy, you dampen inflammation (an important concept I'll define), slow down the aging process, reduce your risk of developing certain diseases, and optimize your biological function.

THE ANATOMY OF AUTOPHAGY

Life is a continual cycle of destruction and building. From the simplest chemistry in which molecules are pulled apart and rearranged to form new compounds, these activities encompass the formation, growth, maintenance, and replication of the cell. They control both single cells and multicellular organisms, from yeast to the human body. Disturb the functioning of either part of this operation—the destruction or the building—too much, and the life process will become dysfunctional and, if not corrected, will eventually end.

As you've already learned, autophagy is a critical biological action in which destruction is utilized within the cell so that its components can be disposed of or recycled in the building process. Compounds or parts of the cell that are "tagged," or marked as defective because they do not fit a certain template (e.g., they are damaged, dysfunctional, or misfolded), are targeted for autophagy. Though you do not have to know all the technical terms of your cellular makeup, I do want you to get a sense of how autophagy works, and it does entail grasping a few key biological concepts.

The cellular events during autophagy follow distinct stages. First, a vesicle precursor, known as the phagophore, is formed. This is a small crescent- or cup-shaped membrane that can sweep up cellular contents as it matures into a spherical double-membraned structure called an autophagosome. Picture a Pac-Man-like structure that engulfs cellular debris that would otherwise gunk up the cell and contribute to inflammatory processes and cause various diseases. Inflammation is the common denominator in all manner of chronic illnesses, from diabetes and heart disease to autoimmune disorders, dementia, and cancer. In small, sporadic episodes, inflammation is the body's survival tool for responding to injury or fighting infection. But many people walk around with chronic inflammation, which the body does not like. Anything that fuels chronic inflammation can lead to ailments rooted in inflammation, which is why cellular debris needs to be cleared out before those inflammatory pathways turn themselves on.

The autophagosome is like a garbage bag or truck, which then fuses with another spherical vesicle called a lysosome that contains enzymes for breaking down (or digesting) many kinds of biomolecules. Lysosomes are like little recycling plants in the body; they are in charge of disposing of waste products and reusing components that are brought in by the garbage trucks. The leftover products from the lysosome's actions are released into the cytoplasm, where they can be reused by the cell. The cytoplasm is the area within a cell that's outside the nucleus. These leftover products include nucleotides, amino acids, free fatty acids, and sugars, which can be used for protein synthesis or oxidized through the mitochondrial electron transport chain to produce energy in the form of adenosine triphosphate, or ATP. The only thing you need to remember about ATP, other than that it's a complex molecule with an equally complex name, is that it gives cells the energy they need to do their work. ATP is the cellular gas that contracts and relaxes our muscles, fires our neurons, and conducts the biochemical reactions necessary to survive. Without the ability to produce ATP, we die.

This process of recycling proteins and lipids helps cells survive under starvation conditions. In fact, the science now says that it is autophagy that actually regulates the function of our cells' mitochondria. This is an important concept to grasp because our mitochondria are indeed "mighty" in ways most people don't appreciate. Your mitochondria are organelles (again, tiny specialized structures) within all of your cells (except red blood cells) that are the source of ATP. They use oxygen within the cell to convert chemical energy from food (e.g., glucose) to energy in a form the cell can use. Put simply, they act like furnaces when they transform glucose into ATP: they "burn" (use) oxygen and give off carbon dioxide and water. Because they generate most of the cell's supply of ATP, they are often referred to as the cell's powerhouse. They have their own DNA, and it's believed that they originated from ancient, so-called proteobacteria. In other words, they were once free-living unicellular organisms that ultimately took up residence within our cells and provided us the ability to produce a new source of chemical energy.*

The human body contains tens of trillions of cells, with an average of 100 mitochondria per cell. Healthy mitochondria are the cornerstone of health and disease prevention. Damaged, dysfunctional mitochondria are linked with every malady imaginable, from autism spectrum disorder to heart disease, diabetes, cancer, dementia, and accelerated aging in general. Not only do you want to stimulate biogenesis to increase mitochondrial numbers, but you need to remove damaged mitochondria via autophagy.

Over the past twenty-five years, researchers have detailed the molecular regulators of the entire autophagy process, which is exquisitely controlled by numerous different signaling pathways. Below is a visual representation of autophagy in action, as cellular debris and toxic materials are swept up for obliteration and recycling.

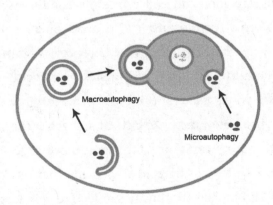

*The origin and evolution of mitochondria are deserving of a book itself. They arose more than 1.45 billion years ago—long before we emerged on the planet. Mitochondria occur in various forms in various multicellular species, plants included. By the time mammals evolved, and eventually we humans, mitochondria had long been part of our biology for generating life-sustaining energy. They are also involved with many other cellular functions, but we won't be getting into those details, as they are tangential to our conversation.

A good question is how much of the cell—and which parts—can be "eaten" without causing it to die. Scientists hypothesize that the level of autophagy and what exactly is obliterated or recycled must be expertly managed to prevent unnecessary cell death and ensure cellular health. When plenty of nutrients are available, for example, the autophagy dial should be turned down, but upon starvation, autophagy must be dialed up. In mammals, autophagy is induced not only by starvation but also by the presence of biological stimuli, such as certain hormones and growth factors, as well as by infection. In general, autophagy is used to sweep up nonspecific components, but it can also selectively degrade damaged cellular parts and bad bacteria that could be harmful. Hence, autophagy likely evolved in the history of life on earth as a shield against the adverse effects of cell starvation. Early on it probably served as a primitive immune defense as well. It does double duty now, preserving life under dangerous conditions of starvation and under ominous conditions of invasion.

Under normal conditions, the process of autophagy occurs continuously at a baseline level, whether a cell is "hungry" or not. It removes faulty proteins and organelles to prevent cell damage. But under stress (e.g., starvation, the absence of growth factors to stir cellular proliferation, or a lack of oxygen), the assembly of players in the autophagy process (phagosomes) increases. Intracellular molecules are then digested to provide the nutrients the cell needs to live. Prolonged autophagy can lead to cell death when too many proteins and organelles essential to the cell's survival are degraded. Clearly, a balance must be struck that likely entails a complex interplay of biochemistry, currently under study. One of the reasons that the relationship between cell death and autophagy sparks researchers' curiosity so much is that they believe autophagy may help treat some of our most dreaded maladies like cancer and neurodegenerative illnesses such as Alzheimer's disease. The magic here is in autophagy's ability to control cell death. Put another way, autophagy could become a therapeutic weapon of sorts, as it protects healthy cells and removes harmful ones.[2]

GUARDIAN OF THE GENOME

One of the first studies to document a link between autophagy and disease was done in 1999. That's when Beth Levine and her colleagues at Columbia University College of Physicians and Surgeons showed that tumors develop after deleting one of the two copies of the cell's Beclin1 gene.[3] Beclin1 is a mammalian version of a gene that is necessary for autophagy. As much as 40 to 75 percent of human breast and ovarian cancers are missing one copy of Beclin1. In Levine's studies, she increased the expression of Beclin1 in human cancer cells, and witnessed more autophagy. When those tinkered cells were injected into mice, the mice developed fewer tumors. Studies done by another team of researchers led by Eileen White at the University of Medicine and Dentistry in New Jersey (now Rutgers Biomedical and Health Sciences) found that autophagy protects against DNA damage.[4] When they inhibited autophagy in experimental mice, they observed more chromosomal abnormalities, which are typically associated with tumor formation. The fact that autophagy can limit DNA damage and chromosomal instability has led scientists to call it the "guardian of the genome."

These discoveries have inspired many scientists around the world to study autophagy's wide spectrum of physiological functions. Researchers have been able to observe how autophagy can promote longevity and benefit virtually every system in the body from the nervous system, immune system, circulatory system, and the metabolism in general. Currently, there are more than 40,000 references on PubMed (the US government's database for life sciences and biomedical scientific papers) about autophagy. Newer findings have linked this cellular process with the prevention of immune and metabolic diseases. The research has been so stunning that autophagy is now being hailed as a center of gravity of sorts for averting diseases such as cancer, neurodegeneration, heart disease, diabetes, liver disease, autoimmune diseases, and infections. There are actually a few different types of autophagy, but the one I just described is the main one used by the body to keep it clean and tidy.

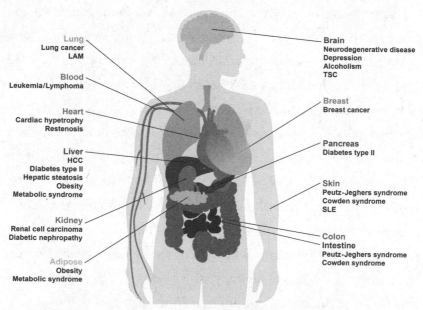

Diseases linked to dysregulated mTOR signaling and the corresponding affected organs. The diseases shown were linked to dysregulated mTOR signaling either by clinical samples from human patients or by genetic disruption of mTOR signaling factors in rodents. For simplicity, diseases are annotated for those organs that are most commonly affected. Tumor syndromes lead to benign tumor growth in multiple organs.

As I noted in chapter 1, we are not the only species to benefit from autophagy. It has been conserved throughout evolution in many plants and animals, including yeast, mold, worms, and flies. Much of what we know about the process has come from studying yeast, mice, and rats. At least thirty-two different autophagy-related genes have been identified by genetic screening studies. We also know that it lies at the heart of survival mechanisms. It's very important in our response to serious threats to our survival, chiefly starvation and stress—and this is true across many species. So it should come as no surprise that if we want to support this process for its antiaging, disease-staving-off properties, we need to employ the twin forces of starvation and stress ever so subtly. And there are ways we can do so within healthy parameters.

AUTOPHAGY'S LIFE-GIVING EFFECTS

Autophagy:

- Recycles damaged proteins, organelles, and other cellular components while defending against misfolded, faulty proteins that can contribute to a number of amyloid-based diseases such as Alzheimer's. Amyloid is a protein that can abnormally build up in certain tissues in the body. It has long been associated with the diseased brain in Alzheimer's patients.

- Provides cells with vital molecular ingredients and energy.

- Regulates the functions of cells' mitochondria, which help produce energy.

- Protects multiple systems in the body to streamline functionality and prevent damage to healthy tissues and organs. In the nervous system, it encourages the growth of brain and nerve cells—ultimately improving cognitive function, brain structure, and the ability of the brain to rewire and reshape itself through new networks ("neuroplasticity"). In the heart, it supports the growth of cardiac cells and protects against heart disease. In the immune system, it helps eliminate potentially harmful pathogens.

- Acts as the "guardian of the genome," protecting the stability of DNA and chromosomes and potentially preventing illnesses such as cancer and neurodegenerative diseases.

Autophaging explains:

- Why cancers and neurological diseases increased dramatically during the twentieth century.

- Why Alzheimer's disease is sometimes called type 3 diabetes.

- What Blue Zones such as Okinawa and Mount Athos have in common and why their residents live long, healthy lives (see chapter 4).

- What bowhead whales and naked mole rats have in common that protects them from cancer (see chapter 8).

- What supercentenarians and the Laron syndrome dwarfs of Ecuador have in common that protects them from cancer (see next chapter).

- Why single gene changes have such a dramatic effect on life span.

- Why certain drugs such as rapamycin, metformin, resveratrol, melatonin, and numerous others that mimic the effects of calorie restriction serve as antiagers.

- Why the consumption of certain antioxidants, such as vitamin E, increases the risk of developing cancer (see chapter 8).

INDUCING AUTOPHAGY NATURALLY

If autophagy is your body's ultimate detoxifying machine for a long, healthy life, you'd certainly want to promote it. And as I just stated, you can do so by placing healthy stressors on your body to boost autophagic processes. Here's how you're going to do that through the two main portals:

Diet

Stick to a high-fat, high-fiber, low-carb diet with minimal protein. Say good-bye to refined carbohydrates and sugars and welcome a bevy of healthy fats and fibrous vegetables. You'll also consider intermittent fasting, which is a powerful trigger for autophagy. Don't panic: I will not ask you to starve yourself. I will make this doable by offering a few ideas for practicing this in real life. You can start with a very comfortable twelve-hour fast just by avoiding eating after 7:00 p.m. (No midnight snacking!) Then you can stretch it to sixteen hours and eventually forgo "breakfast" (breakfast) the next morning, so your first meal of the day is around 11:00.

Intermittent fasting (a form of which is called time-restricted eating) works because it activates the hormone glucagon, which as we learned functions opposite of insulin to keep your blood glucose levels balanced. Although I described this in the previous chapter, here's a visual to really grasp this concept. Picture a seesaw: when one person goes up, the other goes down. This analogy is frequently used to explain the biological insulin-glucagon relationship. In your body, if the insulin level goes up, the glucagon level goes down and vice versa. When you give your body food, your insulin level rises and your glucagon level decreases. But the opposite happens when you don't eat: your insulin level goes down and your glucagon level rises.

When your glucagon level rises, it triggers autophagy. This is why temporarily denying your body nutrients through the safe practice of intermittent fasting (IF) is one of the best ways to boost the integrity of your cells. Aside from maintaining your cells' youth, research has shown that IF promotes greater energy, increased fat burning, and decreased risk of developing diseases such as diabetes and heart disease, all due to its ability to activate autophagy. (See chapter 4 for the full science behind both this type of diet and intermittent fasting.)

Exercise

You already know that exercise does a body good, boosting your metabolism and increasing your cardiorespiratory fitness. But you probably couldn't detail the science of its healthy "stress" on the body to promote autophagy. It actually induces the process in multiple organs that participate in our metabolism, including the liver, pancreas, muscle, and even fat tissue. We often think of exercise as a form of muscle toning and building, but it also breaks down tissues, causing them to be repaired and grow back stronger. In chapter 9, I'll encourage you to start an exercise program even if it's been a while since you last broke a good sweat.

PERIODIC RESTS FROM AUTOPHAGY

As with most everything in life, you'll want to strike a balance between your Switch being on and being off. Exercise is good for you, but it does have its limitations. For instance, if you exercise for long periods of time without rest and at high intensity, the benefits start to dwindle and the liabilities accumulate. Look no further than marathon runners and endurance athletes to understand this law of diminishing returns. They can exhibit signs of heart and kidney damage resulting from ultravigorous levels of exercise for prolonged periods. The same is true of autophagy: the body needs periods of rest from its internal cleansing mechanisms so you can more easily build tissues, keep your weight in check (not lose too much), and maintain your immune system.

In the program outlined in chapter 9, I'll give you some ideas for turning the volume on autophagy down and building your muscles and immune system back up during certain times of the year. You'll want to dial up autophagy for eight months of the year and dial it down during the other four months. It doesn't really matter how you break up those months (e.g., you can do two months with autophagy on and one month off, then repeat for a full calendar year). Remember, autophagy is an action plan or tool for cellular self-fortification, but it also demands a balance as with so many other things in life: too much or not enough can be harmful to the cell, and thus to you.

CHAPTER 3

DWARFS AND MUTANTS

The pace of discovery is going unbelievably fast.
—James Watson (codiscoverer of the structure of DNA)

If I were to ask you what you should be doing to maintain your youth and beauty, increase your healthy life span, and avoid the unwanted side effects of more birthdays, what would you say? Perhaps all of the following:

+ Optimize diet and exercise to sustain ideal weight and physical fitness.

+ Achieve restorative sleep routinely.

+ Manage stress and anxiety.

+ Have chosen parents with longevity genes.

I didn't throw that last bullet point in there just to amuse you. As you know by now, I'm the principal investigator for the Supercentenarian Research Study, which studies the genomics of long-lived humans. Since 2010, I've met and obtained blood samples from sixty people around the world who were 106 years of age and older. The oldest, Emma Morano, of Italy, lived to 117. It's my contention that nearly anyone can live to 100 and maintain robust health by adopting a proper lifestyle—even if you aren't one of the rare individuals who won the genetic lottery. You might be relieved to know that your genes account for much less than you might think when it comes to your life span. Scientists just recently figured this out thanks to analyses of large ancestry databases. It bears reiterating: new calculations show that genes account for well under 7 percent of people's life span—not the 25 to 35 percent of most previous estimates. For the vast majority of us, our longevity is based on our lifestyle choices: what we put in our mouths, how much we move, what kind of stress wears on us, and even other factors such as the quality of our relationships, whom we marry, the strength of our social networks, and our access to health care and education.

The first indication that genes are not the dominant influence came from a study I already mentioned briefly.[1] It entailed more than 400 million people who were born from the nineteenth century to the mid–twentieth century, looking at the life span of spouses. Married couples shared similar life spans—more than siblings did. Such an outcome suggests a strong influence on nongenetic forces because spouses do not typically have genetic variants in common. Other factors that spouses probably do have in common, however, include things such as eating and exercise habits, not smoking, having access to clean water, living far from disease outbreaks, and being literate. This makes sense: people tend to marry others who enjoy the same lifestyles. You don't generally see a couch potato coupled with a triathlete or a party animal married to a teetotaler. And healthy lifestyles make for healthy-behaving genes, or genetic expression.

There's a lot we can learn from individuals who defy the odds of dying and experience healthy lives for a decade or more longer than everyone else. Have you ever wondered, for example, if there is a surefire way to *never* get diabetes or cancer even if you're over-weight or obese? Turns out that there are communities in this world whose members are resistant to those diseases and are pro-tected against some aspects of aging. They may not necessarily live to 100, but they evade two of the most pernicious ailments of modern life that crush millions of people's attempts to live long and well. What secrets do they hold for us?

LARON SYNDROME AND THE ECUADORIANS

As previously mentioned, reducing insulin and IGF-1 levels is related to turning down mTOR and turning up autophagy. Zvi Laron is a physician in Israel (who turned 92 in 2019). His spe-cialty is pediatric endocrinology, which focuses on children with hormonal dysfunctions. In 1958, a Jewish family came to him with three of their young children. The three kids had stunted growth, although there were five older brothers and sisters who were of normal height. Dwarfism, also known as short stature, has many different medical causes, one of which is reduced growth hormone

(GH) production. GH, as you can probably guess, is a substance that stimulates growth, cellular reproduction, and cellular regeneration in humans and other animals. It is made by the pituitary gland at the base of the brain and is so important to development that young adolescents secrete about twice the rate of this hormone per day as adults do (700 micrograms per day versus 400 micrograms per day for adults, mostly during the third and fourth stages of sleep). In addition to helping a young body grow, reach puberty, and mature to adulthood, GH is necessary for strengthening tissues (improving bone density, building muscle) and healing (skin, bones, gut lining, etc.). We produce and use GH throughout our lives, though at varying levels depending on age and needs. Initially, Dr. Laron assumed that this family's unusually small children had a biological shortage of GH, what's called a *deficiency* in medicine, but when he treated them with GH, it didn't seem to help.

Throughout the next decades, more and more short-stature patients sought Dr. Laron's wisdom. Eventually the number of patients reached over sixty, which became known as the "Israeli cohort"; the individuals in this group would go on to be diagnosed with "Laron syndrome," named after Laron's report of the condition together with A. Pertzelan and S. Mannheimer in 1966, based on his experiences with those patients over the years.[2] Adult males with Laron-type dwarfism typically grow to around 4.5 feet tall; women can reach up to 4 feet.

Worldwide, there appear to be between three hundred and five hundred individuals who have this peculiar disorder. In 2014, researchers performing genetic tests to ascertain the genealogical ancestry of Laron syndrome subjects from a half-dozen different countries determined that they were indeed descended from a common ancestor, probably of Jewish descent.[3] Some of that person's descendants stayed in the Middle East or emigrated to eastern Europe; others moved to Spain and Portugal around the second century. Roughly half of the tested Laron syndrome subjects belong to the Sephardic (those from Spain) Jewish group. Following the unification of Spain via the marriage of the "Catholic monarchs" Ferdinand and Isabella in late 1492, the monarchs issued the Alhambra Decree, forcing Jews to either convert to Catholicism or leave the country. Between 40,000 and 100,000 Sephardic Jews left Spain; many settled in northern Africa and the Middle East, but some traveled to other European countries, the Caribbean, South America, and the United States.

In 1987, Dr. Jaime Guevara-Aguirre, an Ecuadorian physician and diabetes expert, began studying a group of about ninety-nine villagers living in the provinces of Loja and El Oro in southern Ecuador, all of whom displayed Laron-type dwarfism. This "Ecuadorian cohort," as they were later known, were descendants of the Sephardic Jews who had fled the Iberian Peninsula and emigrated to Ecuador in the early sixteenth century. Since the Catholic Church was powerful in the major cities such as Lima and Quito, they were forced to settle in more remote southern villages. Fearing persecution, over the next four centuries they remained isolated (their current progeny all live in an area only 150 kilometers in diameter) and because their community was so small, occasionally individuals married close relatives. Why this is important takes us briefly into genetic inheritance models.

GENOTYPES AND PHENOTYPES

Some basic Mendelian genetics will help you understand how characteristics—or, in this case, disorders—are passed on from one generation to the next and end up being common in an isolated geographic area but rare throughout the rest of the world. (Mendelian genetics refers to the laws of inheritance, named after the Augustinian monk Gregor Mendel, who is considered the father of modern genetics. He first established those laws in the 1860s thanks to his experiments with breeding peas in his garden. That was long before we understood DNA, but Mendel documented basic rules of heredity that he gleaned from his observations.)

Your genetic code is found in virtually all of the trillions of cells in your body. It provides the instructions your body needs to operate and carry out basic survival functions. The code is packaged into twenty-three chromosomes, which are like individual volumes of information in the DNA library. The chromosomes are composed of strands of DNA. These strands are arranged in a corkscrew shape, which gives DNA its famous structure that resembles a twisted ladder called a double helix. The rungs of this ladder are made up of about 3 billion base pairs, represented by four chemical bases called nucleotides, which are known most commonly by the letters A (adenine), T (thymine), G (guanine), and C (cytosine). The sequence of these nucleotides forming part of a chromosome are what determine the tens of thousands of genes encoded. As you probably already know, genes are what ultimately dictate everything about you—from the color of your eyes to your risk for developing Alzheimer's or heart disease. It helps to think of the nucleotides as like letters in a special alphabet, and their arrangement creates sentences that govern the expression of your genes.

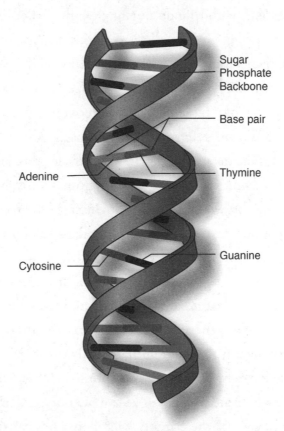

Sugar Phosphate Backbone

Base pair

Adenine

Thymine

Cytosine

Guanine

Our individual characteristics—from what we look like and how fast we can run to nuances in our personality and our risk of developing certain illnesses—are determined largely by the genes we inherit from our parents (yes, environment does play a significant role as well, but for purposes of this discussion, I am focusing purely on genetics). Each of us has about 20,000 to 25,000 genes, but only about 1 percent of these makes you and me the unique individuals we are rather than a generic human. We inherit one set of genes from each parent via the chromosomes. Each genetic character trait is produced by a pair of gene variants called alleles. The individual members of a pair of alleles may be different in their expression, with one dominant over the other. It's purely a matter of chance how these alleles combine and are passed down to the next generation. If you're confused by all this biology jargon, let me simplify this to more practical terms. When a person with blue eyes has biological children with someone who is brown-eyed, the offspring can be a combination of blue- and brown-eyed kids, depending on how the alleles mix and whether or not the brown-eyed parent is passing on a recessive gene for blue eyes. That brown-eyed parent might carry the recessive allele for blue eyes, but it would be masked by the allele for brown eyes, which is dominant.

A mutation in a gene on one of the first 22 non-sex-related chromosomes can lead to a disorder referred to as autosomal. Inherited autosomal genetic mutations are generally either dominant or recessive. If they're dominant, only one copy of the gene from a single parent is required to express the observable characteristics of the disorder (known as the phenotype). In this situation, at least one of the parents will show physical signs of the disorder, i.e., phenotype. A recessive genetic mutation takes place when an abnormal gene (inherited from one parent) is nondominant over the normal gene (inherited from the other parent); the affected individual does not show any outward signs of the abnormal phenotype yet carries a copy of the abnormal gene, which he or she may pass to children (hence he or she is called a carrier of the gene). If the abnormal gene is inherited from both parents, the individual exhibits visible signs. Laron syndrome is one such autosomal recessive disorder.

Autosomal recessive inheritance

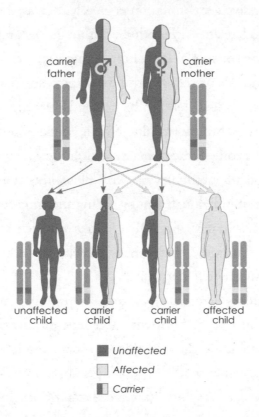

If one of these short-statured individuals has offspring with a person lacking the mutated allele, some of their children may become carriers themselves, but they won't have short stature. If both parents are carriers for the Laron allele—in other words, each of them has only one copy and is unaffected by the disorder—the odds of a biological child also being a carrier is 50 percent; of being a noncarrier, 25 percent; and of expressing the phenotype (having observable signs of the disorder), 25 percent. But if *both* parents express the phenotype (have short stature), that means each must have two copies of the mutated allele and *all* of their children will inherit the dwarfism phenotype. The chance of passing on a recessive gene mutation is greatly increased when people who are blood relatives reproduce. Although generally restricted by social taboos or secular laws, inbreeding occurs more frequently among individuals of certain ethnic backgrounds than others because these individuals tend to be descendants of the same ancestors. In the case of the Sephardic Jews in Ecuador and Israel, their isolation and strong desire to marry within their religion increased the likelihood of intermarrying with close kin, resulting in the high number of individuals among them inheriting the Laron syndrome disorder. In fact, in the first family in which Dr. Laron discovered the syndrome that was named after him, the parents' grandparents were first cousins.

Now, here's where the story gets interesting. Though it may seem like a curse to be born with a genetic destiny for abnormal shortness as an adult, those people also share another uncommon but highly desirable trait: they don't get diabetes or cancer. Ever. They also have a substantially reduced risk of developing Alzheimer's and cardiovascular diseases. What are their biological secrets to being diabetes- and cancer-free for life? Is it their high-altitude village lifestyle, or is it somehow a beneficial side effect of their genetic disorder?

Eight years after Dr. Laron first documented the short-stature kids who were resistant to hormone therapy, a special lab technique called radioimmunoassay became available to measure the growth hormone (GH) level in individuals. Much to his surprise, he found that their GH level was *elevated*, not depressed. He and his colleagues discovered that those kids had a defect in a specific receptor in the liver that is supposed to bind to GH and produce a substance called insulin-like growth factor (IGF-1). Unless you're a biochemist, IGF-1 is not part of your daily vocabulary, but you're going to get to know a lot about this substance because it has everything to do with your longevity—as well as your ability to look and feel great. The blood level of IGF-1 in those who inherited the Laron syndrome mutation from both parents was less than 20 nanograms per milliliter (20 ng/ml). During puberty, the normal range to promote normal development is from 100 to 600 ng/ml; after puberty, the level can range from the 30s to the 200s—much lower than the level needed to meet the body's demands during the growth spurts of maturation. But many adult Americans, due to poor dietary choices, are walking around with high levels that can negatively impact their health. As we'll explore later, too much animal protein and refined carbohydrates will keep IGF-1 levels up.

PROTECTION FROM DIABETES AND CANCER

In 2011, a group of researchers, including Guevara-Aguirre from Ecuador, Rafael de Cabo from the National Institute on Aging, and Valter Longo, a biogerontologist from the University of Southern California Longevity Institute, published a paper showing that after twenty-two years of following the Ecuadorian cohort, there were still no cases of diabetes among them, despite over 20 percent of them being obese and having about the same fasting glucose levels as locals without the mutation.[4] Of the several hundred people in the Ecuadorian cohort, there had been only a single instance of cancer, which had been nonlethal. That was vastly inconsistent with other individuals living in the same area who didn't have the genetic mutation, of whom about 5 percent had died of diabetes and 20 percent of cancer. One of the villagers who continues to be observed in the ongoing study is a woman in her 50s who stands at just three and a half feet tall—the average height of a first grader. She weighs 127 pounds, putting her firmly into the morbidly obese category. Her diet is high in carbohydrates and fats, but her blood pressure is perfect. She has no sign of diabetes or any other illnesses, and despite her obesity, the scientists say that she's healthy.

Earlier Dr. Laron had published a paper in which he and his colleagues had surveyed about one-half (222 individuals) of the world's known population with natural IGF-1 deficiency.[5] Those deficiencies were due to reduced growth hormone, Laron syndrome (because of a mutant growth hormone receptor gene, as just discussed), or the deletion or "loss of function" of the IGF-1 gene. Not one of the individuals presented with a single case of cancer. It didn't even seem to matter that later in life they might have received IGF-1 or GH treatment. When Laron and his colleagues took blood from the Ecuadorian cohort, something in the blood seemed to protect cells grown in a petri dish from laboratory-induced cancers (researchers love to induce cancer in the lab to study its behavior). Despite their high-carbohydrate diet, the Ecuadorian cohort also had reduced insulin levels and good insulin sensitivity (i.e., they were not insulin resistant), which protected them from diabetes (see the box starting on page 59). More important for our concerns, when the researchers incubated human cells in blood from those same people, they had reduced expression of mTOR, the body's chief protein complex, which manages its self-cleansing capabilities. From our previous discussion, you know what that means: with mTOR turned down, autophagy goes up and the cellular recycling machines become activated, clearing out debris and cleaning house.

WHEN AGING GETS STICKY

Insulin is one of the body's most vital hormones, a fact you probably knew already. It plays a starring role in our metabolism, helping us move energy from food into cells for fuel. Because our cells cannot automatically pick up the glucose passing them in the bloodstream, they need the help of insulin, which is produced by the pancreas and acts as a transporter. Insulin transfers glucose from the bloodstream into muscle, fat, and liver cells. Normal, healthy cells have plenty of cellular receptors for insulin and therefore have no problem responding to the hormone. But when cells are relentlessly exposed to high levels of insulin, caused by a constant presence of glucose, they adapt by reducing the number of insulin receptors on their surfaces. They develop a "blind eye" to insulin.

The persistent presence of glucose, by the way, is usually caused by eating too many refined sugars and simple carbs from processed foods. We call this blind-eye effect insulin resistance, as our cells become desensitized, or resistant, to the important hormone. This is believed to be a cellular self-protection mechanism. You see, though glucose can help power cells' energy machinery, called the mitochondria (which we explored in the previous chapters), too much of it can be deadly, sticking to proteins and keeping them from functioning (a process called glycation; more on this below). Once cells are in this state, they ignore insulin and don't pick up glucose from the blood. As with most biological processes, there's a response by the pancreas, which begins to pump out even more insulin. Higher levels of insulin are now required for glucose to enter the cells.

This cascade of events creates a vicious cycle that can eventually culminate in type 2 diabetes. If you're a diabetic, by definition you have hyperglycemia, meaning high (hyper) glucose (gly) in the blood (emia). As a reminder, when you are hyperglycemic, your body has more glucose than needed to immediately power its cells, and the focus becomes storing it safely. First, it's turned into glycogen, a form of glucose that isn't as "sticky" and therefore causes less harm to your cells.

Glycogen is stored mainly in the liver and the muscles, providing the body with a readily available source of energy if the blood glucose level decreases. As long as glycogen stores exist in the liver and muscles, fat will not be burned for fuel and any excess fat consumed will be stored in fat tissue. That may be why most—about 80 percent—of people with type 2 diabetes are overweight or obese. If the sugar remains in the blood, it will inflict a lot of damage, such as the creation of advanced glycation end products (aptly abbreviated AGEs), in which "sticky" glucose molecules attach to proteins (like those that make up your inner blood vessels) and cause dysfunction. Glycation (as the AGE process is called) is part of what makes diabetes a leading cause of early death, coronary heart disease, stroke, kidney disease, and blindness.

What we've learned from the work done by Dr. Laron and others is that there's something about the activity of IGF-1 and its relationship with growth hormone and insulin in the body that affects the risk of developing certain diseases and death. Before we get to a fuller understanding of this, it's important to grasp how we've established a way to study these biological phenomena without experimenting on humans. To do that, we will turn to a few famous mice. All of the previously discussed lessons about genetics and people with short stature may not seem remotely related to autophagy, but they help tell the story, so bear with me. The lessons gleaned from Laron's and others' work have everything to do with how autophagy operates and what we can do to "cheat" our own system's biology to defy the risks of falling ill and dying prematurely.

THE AMES AND SNELL "DWARF" MICE

In the 1950s, at a research mouse colony at Iowa State University in Ames, Iowa, a mouse was born that had a spontaneous mutation in its DNA. This "loss-of-function" mutation in a particular gene resulted in reduced levels of three important hormones: growth hormone, prolactin, and thyrotropin. "Loss of function" simply means that a mutation rendered the gene defunct or inactive—unable to carry out its function, such as coding for proteins that result in the manufacture of certain hormones. Ames dwarf mice look normal at birth, but they grow slowly and reach only about half the size of other members of their family. Adult Ames dwarf mice have extremely low levels of circulating IGF-1. Paradoxically, their food consumption and oxygen utilization are actually higher than what would be expected for their size. Their fasting insulin and glucose levels are also reduced, indicating excellent insulin tolerance (in other words, they are far from being insulin resistant or on the verge of diabetes).

In many respects, Ames dwarf mice have the same delayed aging and longevity benefits displayed by calorie-restricted (CR) animals, without the restriction. Normal mice live on average about 900 days. If you restrict calories in normal mice, they can live as many as 1,200 days. However, Ames dwarf mice live about 1,300 days without calorie restriction and another 100 days longer with calorie restriction.

Like the Ames dwarf mouse, the so-called Snell dwarf mouse has a defect in a different gene that produces certain hormones, including growth hormone. Although there are small differences between these two strains of mice, they have similar pathologies, or biological characteristics. Studies on the unusual longevity of dwarf mice began in the 1990s and early 2000s, many of them conducted by the same researchers who were looking into rapamycin's effects on health span. In one of the first to be published in 2001, David Harrison's eponymous lab at the Jackson Laboratory in Maine, whose work I described in chapter 1, showed that longevity can be extended by the mutations found in both the Snell and Ames dwarf mice.[6] They determined that both have reduced levels of growth hormone and IGF-1. Their work revealed that Snell dwarf mice had delayed aging in certain immune cells and in collagen cross-linking, supporting the conclusion that the extended longevity of this strain of mice is due to authentic deceleration of the rate of aging.

(To be sure, cross-linking refers to a long-established theory of aging whereby certain proteins such as collagen bond together with adverse effects. Diabetics, for instance, have two to three times the numbers of cross-linked proteins as do their healthy counterparts, caused primarily by the high levels of "sticky" glucose in their bloodstream, causing advanced glycation end products, as previously discussed. The cross-linking of proteins may also be responsible for an enlarged heart and the hardening of collagen, which may then lead to an increased susceptibility to cardiac arrest, among other negative outcomes.)

The Snell dwarf mice also had fewer incidences of cancer than normal mice. Dr. Andrezej Bartke, a distinguished scholar and professor of internal medicine and physiology at Southern Illinois University School of Medicine, further proved that supplementing the mice with growth hormone when they were from 2 to 6 weeks old *canceled out* those positive health effects. Dr.

Bartke's laboratory is credited with being among the first to show that a mutation in a single gene can extend mammalian longevity and to suggest that the remarkable increase in the life span of Ames dwarf mice is due to growth hormone (GH) deficiency.[7]

Both the Ames and the Snell dwarf mice strains came about from the spontaneous mutation of a gene that controls the pituitary gland in inbred mice. The GH receptor knockout (GHRKO) mouse strain, on the other hand, was intentionally engineered to re-create the growth hormone receptor defect found in Laron syndrome individuals. Among mice, the GHRKO strain holds the world record for their longevity. This mouse strain was developed to allow researchers to understand this mutation without the ethical and practical limitations of studying it in the human population. These mutant, lab-developed mice exhibit severe growth retardation, proportionate dwarfism, and greatly decreased serum IGF-1 concentration, which duplicates what we see in people with Laron syndrome. Furthermore, GHRKO mice have been found to have decreased fasting glucose and insulin levels and increased insulin sensitivity, as well as decreased glucose tolerance—all beneficial effects in terms of health. And they live 30 to 40 percent longer than their littermates in the wild. In 2017, a consortium of scientists from around the world—from the Mayo Clinic in Minnesota to Brazil, Poland, and Germany—published a paper declaring "a new animal model for aging studies," due to the documented, eye-opening biology of these long-lived mice.[8] Interestingly, centenarians, the best example of successful aging, also have lower plasma IGF-1 levels than do noncentenarians. Numerous animal breeds (e.g., miniature and teacup dogs, cats, and pigs), whose dwarfish size is due to a single mutation in their IGF-1 gene, also live remarkably longer than do their normal-sized counterparts.

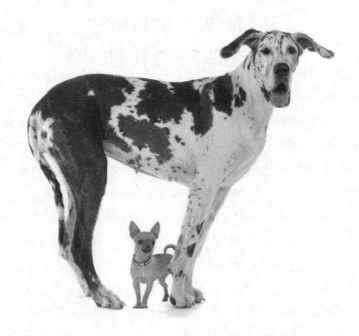

My whole point in outlining the evolution of lab mice that live relatively longer than their mutant-free counterparts is to show that we now have a way of studying these unique mutations to understand where in the body's machinery we can make certain tweaks to bestow longevity—and, more important, how we can mimic the effects of these mutations through basic lifestyle interventions. Having a lower level of IGF-1 equates with having a longer life. But you don't need to have a mutant gene to achieve these results. Interestingly, calorie restriction—the most reproducible intervention to extend animal life span—will substantially reduce your IGF-1 level. The key is to strike a healthy balance and respect

IGF-1's relationship with growth hormone and insulin to optimize aging and autophagy.

THE TRADE-OFF BETWEEN PERFORMANCE AND LONGEVITY

As just mentioned, growth hormone (GH) has numerous effects on the body, both on tissue growth and on energy metabolism. GH is released in response to a variety of situations or circumstances, the most important of which for our purposes are exercise, a decrease in blood glucose, and carbohydrate restriction or fasting. As previously defined and as its name suggests, GH is a growth-promoting hormone, increasing protein synthesis in the muscle and liver. GH also tends to marshal free fatty acids from fat cells for energy, a key component of weight loss.

Here's an important fact that I've left out until now: I said that GH stimulates the liver to produce IGF-1, but it does so *only in the presence of insulin*. A high GH level along with a high insulin level (for instance, after eating a meal that contains protein and carbohydrates, such as a pepperoni pizza or cheeseburger) will raise the IGF-1 level as well as increase growth-promoting reactions in the body. To the contrary, a high GH level with a low level of insulin, as seen during fasting or carbohydrate restriction, will not cause an increase in the IGF-1 level and has many beneficial effects. By stimulating autophagy, we can clear out all our old, useless, and potentially harmful proteins and cellular debris. At the same time, fasting stimulates growth hormone, which tells our body to start producing some snazzy new cells and tissues. We are boosting the health of our bodies through a continuous and complete renovation: out with the old, in with the new. It's similar to renovating a room in your house, say your kitchen: if dilapidated 1960s-style avocado green cabinets are on your walls, you need to remove them before you can install new ones. It's a dual process of removal or destruction and creation or building.

Clearly, there is a time and place for promoting growth in the body and having a certain level of IGF-1 circulating. Having either a too-low or too-high IGF-1 level increases the risk of dying of all-cause mortality (meaning dying of any disease). On the one hand, IGF-1 promotes development and is therefore important for recovery purposes, but that same mechanism means it can promote cancer. Here is a summary of IGF-1's pros and cons:

Some of the Pros

+ Helps maintain muscle mass and strength, reducing muscle wasting and overall fragility

+ Reduces inflammatory responses and suppresses oxidative stress

+ Enhances cell survival in the face of hazards, including DNA damage

+ Boosts brain health by triggering the growth of new neurons, preventing the accumulation of amyloid plaques, and acting as a natural anti-depressant

+ Protects against heart disease by having anti-inflammatory and antioxidant effects on blood vessels, stabilizing existing plaque, and reducing additional plaque accumulation

+ Helps increase bone density

+ Supports the immune system

The Big Cons

+ Heightens the risk of developing cancerous growths; IGF-1 is a cancer promoter

+ Shortens life span

Say what? How is this possible? I listed multiple positive effects of IGF-1 signaling and just two, albeit significant, cons. In scientific circles, this conundrum is called the IGF-1 paradox: despite the cell proliferation and survival-enhancing properties attributed to IGF-1, it is a reduction in IGF-1 signaling that has been shown to extend life span in multiple organisms including nematodes, flies, and mammals. This is an area of active study today. One of the theories behind the paradox being explored is the role of the mitochondria, the tiny organelles in our cells that generate chemical energy in the form of ATP. Mitochondria, you'll recall, are the workhorses of our cells; they are found in all cells except red blood cells and have their own DNA separate from the DNA in the nuclei. We now think that they take a major part in the development of degenerative diseases such as Alzheimer's, Parkinson's, and cancer. In fact, mitochondrial diseases include a group of neurological, muscular, and metabolic disorders caused by dysfunctional mitochondria. Disorders as diverse as diabetes and dementia have all been linked to mitochondrial problems.[9] Anytime there is mitochondria damage or dysfunction, disease and aging follow.

Here's the key point: Autophagy may play an important role in the normal turnover of mitochondria. When the level of IGF-1 is continually high, mTOR is turned on and autophagy is turned off, leading to mitochondrial dysfunction and decreased cell viability. And because mitochondrial mutations and dysfunction may naturally increase with age, the reduced clearance of dysfunctional mitochondria in settings in which the IGF-1 level is elevated may be significant in age-related ailments and conditions.[10]

HOW TO ACTIVATE THE BODY'S BUILT-IN ANTIAGING MOLECULE

One of the safest and most effective methods of optimizing autophagy is by activating an enzyme recently discovered in our cells called 5' ("five-prime") adenosine monophosphate-activated protein kinase (AMPK), known more colloquially as the body's natural antiaging enzyme. When AMPK is activated, it tells cells to remove internal pollutants via autophagy. This enables cells to act in a more youthful manner, as evidenced by reduced abdominal fat stores in many people using AMPK-activating compounds (AMPK signals cells to devour internal fat, among other substances). The popular diabetes drug metformin, in fact, works by decreasing the production of ATP in the mitochondria, which stimulates AMPK activity, thereby resulting in greater insulin sensitivity. As we might expect, IGF-1 actions are turned down when AMPK is signaling. We also know that AMPK may turn on our "antioxidant genes," which are responsible for our body's natural production of antioxidants. The following three strategies will help you activate this vital antiager, and they will be part of the program outlined later.

- Exercise, especially high-intensity interval training

- Dietary inputs: viscous dietary fiber such as that found in whole fruits and vegetables, as well as legumes (e.g., beans, lentils); polyphenol-rich teas such as green tea; and curcumin, the active compound found in turmeric

- Calorie restriction with intermittent fasting and protein restriction (see next chapter)

TIMING IS EVERYTHING

As the saying goes, in life, timing is everything. And as with so many facets of life, there is a good side and a bad side to reconcile. We need IGF-1 for survival to some degree, just as our body requires inflammation, cholesterol, and body fat at the appropriate times and in the appropriate amounts. But get too much of anything, and, well, trouble arises. We must strive to keep all of these biological events or substances in balance and leverage their power when we need them most. When we're young and developing and our risk of cancer is relatively low, IGF-1 is a friend to have around for superior growth and development, as well as for recovery from injury. Certain other circumstances can also call for keeping IGF-1 signaling on, such as during pregnancy and lactation.* But as we get older, the scales tip in the other direction and we would do well to start curbing our IGF-1 signaling—especially as we approach midlife and cancer risk begins to climb

---

*Pregnancy and lactation are just two of many circumstances that can call for keeping IGF-1 signaling on. Speak with your doctor if you have any unique conditions to consider.

dramatically with natural cellular aging and the accumulation of DNA mutations in our cells. Our modern diets, which are rich in refined carbs and animal proteins, do not help, further making the case for following a monk's diet to turn the volume down on IGF-1 and favor autophagy. We will discuss this more in subsequent chapters.

There's a sound biological reason why high animal protein diets increase the risk of developing cancer. And that reason relates to IGF-1. You see, when we bombard the body with lots of protein, our liver responds with a call to do something productive with it all and pumps out IGF-1 to essentially tell cells, "It's growing time! Start your engines and multiply—we've got a lot of extra protein to work with and make things."

The problem is that some of the additions spurred by this growth hormone may be tumors, especially if autophagy has been turned off too long and you have lots of dysfunctional mitochondria producing mutagenic free radicals that have further damaged your cells' DNA. When you're a fully grown adult, cell growth is something you want to slow down, not accelerate (despite what the peddlers of pro-growth "antiaging" hormones and supplements would have you believe). The goal therefore is to maintain adequate, but not excessive, overall protein intake. And I'm referring chiefly to animal proteins; plant-based proteins have far less of the amino acids that increase levels of IGF-1. Which is why the Mediterranean diet combined with intermittent fasting is ideal for managing this balancing act.

As we'll see in the next chapter, the Greek Orthodox monks of Mount Athos are among the healthiest people on Earth. Research has repeatedly shown that within their tight-knit communities cancer is almost unheard of, strokes and cardiac arrests are pretty much nonexistent, and diseases such as Alzheimer's and Parkinson's are extremely rare. The monks have also been proven to live, on average, several years longer than men living in mainland Greece. Indeed, their lifestyle holds a few surprising secrets for us to heed.

CHAPTER 4

OKINAWANS, MONKS, AND SEVENTH-DAY ADVENTISTS

Everyone has a physician inside him or her; we just have
to help it in its work. The natural healing force within
each one of us is the greatest force in getting well. Our food
should be our medicine. Our medicine should be our food.
But to eat when you are sick is to feed your sickness.

—Hippocrates

What do some Okinawans, Greeks, and Seventh-Day Adventists have in common? Like those Laron syndrome dwarfs, they enjoy long, disease-free lives by keeping the process of autophagy actively running inside their cells in healthy harmony. How do they do this? Let's explore these three remarkable groups of people who inhabit the same planet as we do but outpace our performance in how long and how well they live. By examining their lifestyles, we can garner the secrets of their success and implement them in our own lives. This entails an exploration of three biological marvels on the body:

+ Calorie restriction

+ Intermittent fasting

+ Protein cycling

First we'll look at the Okinawans, who give us clues to the benefits of reducing both our protein and calorie intake.

FEWER CALORIES, LONGER LIFE

Okinawa is the largest of the chain of islands that form Japan's southernmost prefecture (similar to a state or province). It lies almost a thousand miles south of Tokyo and has a subtropical climate. The citizens of Okinawa are noted for having the longest life expectancy within Japan (and likely the world), mainly because they avoid or delay major age-associated diseases such as diabetes, heart disease, stroke, and cancer. They have the lowest rates of these ailments globally. Japan's population is only 40 percent that of the United States, but the country currently has more living supercentenarians who have surpassed the 110-year mark. The oldest person ever from Japan was Misao Okawa, who died in 2015 at the age of 117 in Osaka on the mainland, where she was born in 1898. On her 117th birthday—about a month before her death of heart failure—she said that her life seemed short. When asked about the secret of her longevity, she replied, jokingly, "I wonder about that, too."

Okinawans age slowly and get heart disease at only 20 percent the rate of Westerners. According to Drs. Bradley and Craig Willcox, brothers who work with the now-famous Okinawa Centenarian Study, begun in the 1970s by Dr. Makoto Suzuki, breast cancer is so rare that screening mammography isn't routinely needed, and most aging men don't talk or even worry about prostate cancer.[1] On average, they spend 97 percent of their lives free of any disabilities. But studies suggest that when they emigrate, to either Japan's mainland or Hawaii, for example, they quickly lose their health advantages, meaning that their longevity is not strongly linked to genetics. Not uncoincidentally, Okinawa is Japan's poorest region. For decades, the custom there was to eat only until one felt 80 percent full. Whether this was cultural or just being frugal out of necessity, Okinawans traditionally consumed 20 percent fewer calories than did adults on the Japanese mainland.

There are multiple aspects attributed to the longevity of the Okinawan elders: physical activity through martial arts, walking, gardening, and traditional Okinawan dance; spirituality and stress reduction; social support; and a good health care system. But diet is the foundation of their success.[2] As described by the Okinawa Centenarian Study's Craig Willcox, a medical anthropologist and gerontologist, the traditional dietary pattern in this region of Japan has the following characteristics:

1. High consumption (about 73% of total calories) of low-glycemic vegetables, such as nonstarchy vegetables (e.g., artichokes, asparagus, avocados, broccoli, cabbage,

cauliflower, celery, cucumbers, greens, mushrooms, onions, peppers, spinach, summer squash, tomatoes, zucchini). The glycemic index (GI) was developed almost forty years ago as a measure of how foods, particularly carbohydrate-containing foods, influence the amount of glucose in the blood. The GI uses a scale of 0 to 100, and it uses pure glucose as the reference point to assign values to certain foods. Pure glucose has a GI of 100. Foods with a high GI (generally 70+) are rapidly digested and absorbed. This causes a fast elevation in the blood sugar level, which in turn triggers a spike in the level of insulin, the hormone responsible for ushering glucose out of the bloodstream and into cells for use. Low-GI foods (generally those with a value of 1 to 55) are digested more slowly, producing gradual rises in blood sugar and insulin levels. Some low-GI foods change blood sugar levels hardly at all. Foods with a GI value of 56 to 69 are considered "medium."

2. High consumption of legumes, mostly in the form of tofu and miso (soy paste). The tofu in Okinawa is lower in water content than the Japanese version and higher in healthy fat and protein.

3. Moderate consumption (about 1% of daily calories) of fish products, especially in coastal areas.

4. Low consumption (less than 1% of daily calories) of meat and meat products.

5. Low consumption (less than 1% of daily calories) of dairy products.

6. Moderate alcohol consumption.

7. Low calorie intake.

8. High consumption of omega-3 fats from fish.

9. High monounsaturated-to-saturated-fat ratio.

10. Emphasis on low-GI carbohydrates in general.

To these I would add:

11. Low consumption (less than 1% of daily calories) of fruit.

12. Low consumption (about 39 grams a day) of protein.

13. High consumption (about 23 grams a day) of fiber.

The especially low protein content of the traditional Okinawan meal is a drastic enough protein restriction to turn off mTOR and substantially reduce IGF-1 levels.

Notable is the high intake of vegetables, particularly sweet potatoes and soy, and few meat or dairy products as their main sources of protein. The Okinawan sweet potato, which has a low caloric density, was the main carbohydrate of the Okinawan diet from the 1600s until approximately 1960, accounting for more than 50 percent of calories. (Although you'd think it would be high on the glycemic index, it's nothing compared to a baked white potato, which comes in at around 85; a boiled sweet potato has a GI value in the mid-40s and has fewer carbs and calories.) When the Okinawa Centenarian Study researchers measured the DHEA levels of octogenarians on the island and compared them to a US reference population in Rancho Bernardo, a community in the northern hills of San Diego, California, they documented higher levels of the hormone among the Okinawans. Not to be confused with the omega-3 fatty acid docosahexaenoic acid (DHA), dehydroepiandrosterone (DHEA) is a hormone that is made by the human body. It is manufactured by the adrenal glands and is one of the most abundant circulating hormones, serving as a precursor of other hormones, such as estrogen and testosterone. DHEA falls steadily as we age and is therefore a good biomarker of how fast a person is aging. The Okinawans were also found to have higher levels of natural estrogen and testosterone than Americans of the same age. A healthy diet and continual physical activity are thought to explain why these hormones remain so high in elderly Okinawans.

If diet is the main secret of the Okinawans' long, disease-free life, which of their dietary habits is the "it" factor? Of all the features just enumerated, one stands out: calorie restriction (CR), now established to be the most powerful intervention to delay aging and increase longevity in diverse species, from yeast to mammals. It is also the most potent and reproducible physiological intervention to protect against cancer specifically in mammals. The idea that organisms can live longer, healthier lives by sharply reducing their calorie intake is not new science. Studies involving the life span and health benefits of calorie restriction have been published and reviewed extensively ever since the publication in 1935 of renowned Cornell University nutritionist Clive McCay's seminal paper with Mary Crowell and Leonard Maynard in *The Journal of Nutrition*, cited thousands of times in the past several decades.[3] McKay's team was the first to demonstrate that simply reducing calorie intake without causing malnutrition nearly doubled the life span of rats. Their research established a foundation for future studies showing that aging can be slowed down. Nearly half a century later, Richard Weindruch and Roy Walford reported that "adult-initiated" calorie restriction beginning at 12 months of age in rats—the equivalent of a thirty-year-old human—not only increased the life span of rats but also reduced their incidence of spontaneous cancer by more than 50 percent.[4] Several decades later, laboratory research has repeatedly demonstrated the anti-aging value of calorie restriction in animals from worms and flies to rodents and primates—with the strong implication that the same should be true for our species of primate. The benefits documented across various forms of life points to a highly conserved effect, evolutionarily speaking, that likely involves common genes.

The Okinawans—prior to coming under the dietary influences of Western cultures (after World War II, the United States operated military bases there, employing tens of thousands of personnel and their families, bringing American grocery stores, diners, and fast food)—were models of calorie restriction. Previous to that, they had consumed about 1,780 calories daily—11 to 15 percent fewer than would normally be recommended to maintain their body weight. (A typical adult diet on a normal day includes about 2,000 calories.) Younger Okinawans who did not follow a CR diet had higher body mass indexes (BMIs) at all ages, as well as a higher incidence of type 2 diabetes and a higher risk of developing heart disease.

By definition, calorie restriction involves the consumption of fewer calories *without malnutrition* or deprivation of essential nutrients. This triggers many biological effects on the body that ultimately mimic the longevity benefits of a drug such as rapamycin (discussed in chapter 1). Although the molecular mechanisms that control the effects of calorie restriction are still being studied and debated, there is more widespread acceptance of the hypothesis that calorie restriction and life span extension involve a dialing down of insulin signaling and a dialing up of autophagy.

In 2017, a collaborative group of researchers, including some from the University of Wisconsin–Madison and the National Institute on Aging, reported in the journal *Nature* that chronic calorie restriction promotes measurable health benefits in the rhesus monkey—a primate with a humanlike aging pattern—indicating "that CR mechanisms are likely translatable to human health."[5] The researchers, one of whom was Dr. Weindruch of earlier fame, described one monkey they started on a 30 percent calorie restriction diet when he was 16 years old, which is late middle age for this type of animal. The rhesus monkey (named Canto) is now well over forty, a longevity record for the species, and the equivalent of a human living past 130.

In another recent study led by USC's Valter Longo, whom I first introduced in chapter 3, his team suggested that it's possible to gain antiaging benefits without committing to a lifetime of chronic hunger. He recommends what he calls a "fasting-mimicking diet," practiced just five days a month for three months and repeated at intervals as needed. Professor Longo states that such a protocol is "safe, feasible and effective in reducing risk factors for aging and age-related diseases."[6]

In Longo's study, people followed a carefully designed protocol that entailed a 50 percent calorie-restricted diet (totaling about 1,100 calories) on the first day and a 70 percent calorie-restricted diet (about 700 calories) on the next four days, after which they could eat whatever they wanted for the rest of the month. According to Longo, the underlying theory of this protocol is that the regenerative effects of the regimen occur during the recovery period after the fast. Such a protocol, even for just five days, is not for everyone. It was hard enough on Longo's test subjects to result in a dropout rate of 25 percent. But for those who stuck with it, especially people who were obese or otherwise unhealthy, multiple benefits were documented. After the third month, participants experienced decreased body mass (without the loss of lean muscle mass) and healthier levels of blood sugar, blood fats, and cholesterol. Best of all, these results remained for at least three more months—even after they had returned to a normal diet full-time.

By choice, various people have practiced extreme degrees of calorie restriction over many years. These individuals do so in the belief that it will extend their life span or somehow preserve their health. As outlined by the National Institute on Aging, studies of these individuals have found markedly low levels of risk factors for certain ailments, such as cardiovascular disease and diabetes. But these benefits may come at a cost. The studies have also found many other physiological effects whose long-term benefits and risks are uncertain, as well as reduced libido and reduced ability to maintain body temperature in a cold environment. These people generally consume a variety of nutritional supplements, which limits being able to determine which effects are due to calorie restriction as opposed to other factors. So you can rest assured that a safe practice like that of the Okinawans is sufficient; you don't have to take CR to extremes. There is a law of diminishing returns to respect.

To conduct a more rigorous study of calorie restriction in humans, the National Institute on Aging (NIA) is supporting a pioneering clinical trial under the stewardship of Duke University School of Medicine called Comprehensive Assessment of Long-Term Effects of Reducing Intake of Energy (CALERIE).[7] This is an ongoing study being carried out at the Pennington Biomedical Research Center in Baton Rouge, Louisiana, the Jean Mayer USDA Human Nutrition Research Center on Aging at Tufts University in Boston, and the Washington University in St. Louis School of Medicine in Missouri. Although the study remains in motion, we already have some data from trials that have concluded since it began in 2007. The study recruited 218 young and middle-aged, normal-weight or moderately overweight adults who were randomly divided into two groups. People in the experimental group were told to follow a calorie restriction diet for two years, while those in the control group followed their usual diet.

The study was designed to have those in the experimental group eat 25 percent fewer calories per day than they had regularly consumed before the study. Although they did not meet the target due to the difficulty of cutting back so much, the participants managed to reduce their daily calorie intake by 12 percent and reap benefits. The subjects maintained, on average, a 10 percent loss in body weight over two years. Importantly, a follow-up study two years after the intervention ended found that the subjects had sustained much of their weight loss.

I'd like to reiterate here that a calorie restriction regimen is not a starvation diet. The weight loss recorded with calorie restriction in the CALERIE trial was still within the normal or even overweight range. But they showed reduced risk factors for many health conditions. Compared to participants in the control group, those in the calorie restriction group had reduced risk factors (lower blood pressure and lower LDL cholesterol level) for age-related diseases such as diabetes, heart disease, and stroke. They also experienced decreases in some inflammatory factors and thyroid hormones (more on the thyroid connection shortly). There is some evidence that lower levels of these are associated with longer life span and a decreased risk of developing age-related diseases. And in the calorie-restricted individuals, no negative effects were found on quality of life, mood, sexual function, and sleep.

The calorie restriction intervention did cause slight declines in bone density, lean body mass (i.e., muscle), and aerobic capacity (the ability of the body to use oxygen during exercise). But those declines were generally no more than expected based on the subjects' weight loss. Other short-term studies have found that combining physical activity with calorie restriction protects against losses of bone, muscle mass, and aerobic capacity. That's another clue we need to heed: exercising helps cancel out any potential adverse effects of the restricted calorie intake. I should also add that the CALERIE group continues to be evaluated by various researchers around the world. In 2019, for example, a team from Brazil and Canada concluded that the CR of healthy participants over those two years had led to positive effects on working memory compared to the control subjects, who ate whatever they wanted. Such a result "opens new possibilities to prevent and treat cognitive deficits," the authors of that study wrote.[8]

What's going on in the body when it's deprived of an abundance of calories? And what's the key to cutting back without feeling deprived? We'll get to the second question later. For now, let's address the first one.

The effects of calorie restriction on growth hormone, and in turn levels of insulin and IGF-1, are certainly important to keeping your "growth" switch (mTOR) tuned down so that your self-cleaning process (autophagy) is tuned up. You'll recall that Dr. Andrezej Bartke's dwarf mice that lived much longer than their normal counterparts could attribute their longevity to growth hormone deficiency. This ties directly into autophagy. With less growth hormone around, there's increased autophagy to clean house. And what's the relationship between calorie restriction and autophagy? When you put mild stress on the body in the form of calorie restriction, it turns up the autophagy dial. As that happens, there's an increase in protein turnover and cellular repair. In other words, your body is forced to renovate itself! Just as you'd tear out old appliances in a kitchen remodel before bringing in new ones and painting, the same type of process takes place in the body. Certain proteins and tissues are destroyed so new ones can form to replace them. This is the essence of autophagy.

One of the most compelling theories of aging, in fact, revolves around a lack of protein turnover; if the body cannot break down and dispose of old protein as it builds new protein, damaged protein will accumulate and start to wreak havoc (note that this does not apply only to muscles; protein is everywhere in your body, from your heart to your skin). Balanced protein turnover is critical, and it's spurred by calorie restriction.

A number of studies using laboratory animals have focused on CR's effects. Calorie restriction affects many processes that have been proposed to control the rate of aging. These include inflammation, glucose metabolism, maintenance of protein structures, the capacity to provide energy for cellular processes, and modifications to DNA. Another important process that is affected by calorie restriction is oxidative stress, which is the production of toxic by-products (called free radicals) of oxygen metabolism that can damage cells and tissues. Free radicals, which I'm sure you've heard about before, are like rogue atoms in the body that can be harmful when they accumulate and are not countered by antioxidants.

Many of the processes I just mentioned were similarly affected by calorie restriction in the human CALERIE trial. As the study participants dialed down their calorie intake, their bodies dialed up autophagy with resulting benefits, including a general deceleration of aging. A general rule that many experts in this area of medicine agree on is to eat 15 percent less starting at age 25. Such a reduction might add 4.5 healthy years to your life, according to Dr. Eric Ravussin, who studies human health and performance at the Pennington Biomedical Research Center in Baton Rouge and was among the scientists who led the CALERIE study.[9]

Another study worth mentioning was done by Edward Weiss and his colleagues at Saint Louis University.[10] They studied men and women aged 50 to 60 who did not smoke, were not obese, and were in good health but relatively sedentary. The volunteers were split into three groups—a calorie restriction group, an exercise group, and a control group—and followed for one year. The calorie restriction group cut back by 300 to 500 calories per day (if you're wondering how you can do this easily, see the box starting on page 89). Volunteers in the exercise group maintained their usual diet and exercised regularly. Though both the calorie restriction and exercise groups experienced similar changes in body fat mass, only those in the calorie restriction group experienced lower thyroid hormone levels.

A low thyroid hormone level sounds like a bad thing, and many people take supplemental thyroid hormones to correct for thyroid dysfunction that can lead to hypothyroidism, or an under-performing thyroid. An overactive thyroid, or hyperthyroidism, is also possible, but the former is much more common. To be sure, thyroid hormones, which are produced by the thyroid gland at the base of the neck, are important for a wide variety of biological functions. They are responsible for growth, metabolism rate, and energy expenditure and help to maintain cognition and bone and cardiovascular health. This is why any dysfunction of the thyroid gland and its output can be harmful to your health. Now, here's what's intriguing: it turns out that some forms of reduced thyroid function tend to be associated with increased longevity in a number of species. And a predisposition to a low thyroid hormone level appears to be inherited in long-lived families. Researchers suggest that the lower thyroid hormone activity could shift the body's energy expenditure away from growth and proliferation in favor of protective maintenance (autophagy), keeping the body healthier longer. Another explanation for the benefits of lower levels of thyroid hormones relates to there being less oxidative stress on the body. An important point is that "reduced" function doesn't mean "out of the normal range." You can have low thyroid function within the normal range to reap both the benefits of a healthy thyroid on the body and an increased chance for a longer life.

Dr. Weiss continues to devote his research to documenting the benefits of CR and exercise, especially when used together. In some of his more recent work, his lab has found that the combination of CR and exercise boosts metabolism—particularly glucose regulation and insulin sensitivity—much more than either of those interventions alone, even when the weight loss is the same.[11] I'll help you find a CR regimen you can stick to in the program outlined in chapter 9. For now, let's turn to a few long-lived monks.

HOW TO EASILY CREATE A DEFICIT OF 500 CALORIES A DAY

1. Skip the bread; have a salad instead of a sandwich.

2. Swap soda for water.

3. Drink your coffee black with no sweeteners or other added sugars (and no blended coffees).

4. Cook your meals at home. When you order in, dine out, or heat up premade meals, you consume a lot more calories (as well as overprocessed ingredients).

5. Slow down when you eat. Doing so will enable you to consume up to 300 fewer calories per meal, according to a

study in the *Journal of the American Dietetic Association.*
In the course of a day, your savings will be well over 500
calories.[12]

6. Work out before breakfast. A 2015 Japanese study found
that when you exercise before breakfast, you metabolize
about 280 more calories throughout the day, compared
with doing the same workout in the evening.[13] Add that
to a rule of not eating after 7:00 p.m., and you'll rack up
a saving of 520 calories. A study published in the *British Journal of Nutrition* in 2013 revealed that eliminating
nighttime snacks helped people consume 240 fewer calories daily.[14]

7. Put away your phone during meals. According to a study
published in *The American Journal of Clinical Nutrition,*
people who looked at their phone during lunch, whether to
peruse social media, trawl the internet in general, or lose
themselves in a game, tended not to remember their meal
well, felt less full, and snacked more in the afternoon—and
they consumed about 200 more calories a day.[15]

LIVE (LONG) LIKE A MONK

Some Greek monks have virtually no cancer, heart disease, or Alzheimer's disease. They also live about a decade longer than the average Greek. Who are these people? They are a group of approximately two thousand Greek Orthodox monks living in about twenty monasteries on Mount Athos, a mountainous peninsula in northeastern Greece. Life on Mount Athos has changed little over the past millennia. Much of the monks' day is taken up with chores: cleaning, cooking, and tending to vegetable gardens. Since 1994, the monks have been tested regularly, and only eleven have developed prostate cancer, one-quarter the international average. Lung and bladder cancer are nonexistent.

According to Greek mythology, the giant Athos threw a rock at Zeus, who knocked it to the ground near Macedonia, the peak of which became the holy peak of Mount Athos. Though it is connected to the mainland of Greece, it consists of a long peninsula with steep sides, surrounded by turbulent seas. In the fifth century BCE, the Greek historian Herodotus wrote about the Persians' losing three hundred ships and twenty thousand men in a storm just off the coast of Mount Athos, causing the Persian general Mardonius to retreat back into Asia Minor. In 411 BCE, the Spartans lost fifty ships to those dangerous seas. To this day, the peninsula remains accessible practically only by ferry.

According to tradition, the Virgin Mary, following Christ's death, was sailing with Saint John the Evangelist toward Cyprus to visit Lazarus. Caught in a sudden storm, their boat was blown off course to the Mount Athos peninsula. Mary walked ashore and was immediately overwhelmed by the beauty of the land. She blessed the island and asked her son Jesus to give it to her as a garden. Legend has it that a voice was heard saying "Let this place be your inheritance and your garden, a paradise and a haven of salvation for those seeking to be saved." From then on, no women were to be allowed there, out of respect for the Virgin Mary.

Monks are thought to have arrived on Mount Athos in about

the third century. One legend has it that women were banned by them because the monks became too frisky with shepherdesses; another legend claims that after several monks reported having had visions of the Virgin Mary, it was decided that the monks should devote themselves to her and that no other woman should be allowed to outshine her. Since at least the ninth century, this self-governing state of Greece has been proclaimed a holy place of monks, and admission to the island has been limited to males. Even now, the number of daily visitors is limited, and women remain prohibited. It is the only UNESCO World Heritage Site recognized for both its cultural (there are religious art works and texts going back a thousand years) and its natural significance.

The monks of Mount Athos hold many secrets, and among the most talked about—besides the region's storied, somewhat mythical past—is their extraordinary good health, which has been largely attributed to their dietary habits, similar to the Okinawans'. The monks eat two Mediterranean diet–style meals a day. Both meals last only ten minutes. Breakfast is just hard bread and tea. The evening meal contains some fish, bread, legumes, home-grown fruits and vegetables, and red wine (dairy products and eggs are supplied from surrounding areas, since animal husbandry and poultry farming are prohibited; but the monks do eat cheese and eggs). Some of the seaside monasteries specialize in catching octopus, a delicacy that is softened by bashing it on the rocks. Fish also feed the Mount Athos cats, protected by the monks for their mouse-catching prowess (female cats are the only females intentionally allowed on Mount Athos; the no-female policy is what prohibits animal husbandry and poultry farming).

Three days a week, the monks fast, eating a vegan diet. Fasting in the Greek Orthodox Church means abstaining from meat, some types of fish, dairy products (milk, cheese, and yogurt), oil, and wine. Only on rare feast days do the monks have sweets, such as cake or ice cream, and even then only in moderation. Orthodox Christian holy books recommend a total of 180 to 200 days of fasting per year.

A Greek researcher, Katerina Sarri at the University of Crete, has looked at the effects of Greek Orthodox fasting on blood fat levels and obesity.[16] She compared sixty subjects who fasted around the high holy seasons of the year—forty days before Christmas, forty-eight days during Lent, and fifteen days before the Feast of the Assumption—with similar Greek adults who didn't practice fasting. She characterized the Greek Orthodox fasts as requiring a periodic vegetarian diet, including some seafood, since seafood such as shrimp, squid, cuttlefish, octopus, lobsters, and crabs, as well as snails (all of which are without "backbones"), are allowed on all fasting days throughout the year. The people who fasted had 12 percent lower total cholesterol and 16 percent lower LDL levels, compared to the nonfasters. Their HDL level was slightly lower, but their LDL/HDL ratios were better.

Intermittent fasting, sometimes referred to as time-restricted feeding, has a long history dating back thousands of years (there's a reason why most religions incorporate fasting into their practice). As you can likely guess, there's an overlap between the practice of fasting and calorie restriction because fasting in itself results in calorie restriction. And some protocols, such as those of Dr. Longo described previously, entail a blend of fasting on some days and reducing calories on others.

Hippocrates, a Greek physician who lived in the fifth and

fourth centuries BCE, was one of the fathers of Western medicine, from whom we inherited the Hippocratic Oath. Among his writings, he proposed that both disease and epilepsy could be treated with complete abstinence from food and drink. A Greco-Roman philosopher, Plutarch, in a work entitled "Advice about Keeping Well," said, "Instead of using medicine, rather fast [for] a day." Avicenna, a great Arab physician, often prescribed fasting for three weeks or more.

The ancient Greeks used fasting and calorie-restricted diets to treat epilepsy. The Greek physician Erasistratus declared, "One inclining to epilepsy should be made to fast without mercy and be put on short rations," and Galen, the famed Greek physician and surgeon who practiced in the Roman Empire in the second century CE, recommended an "attenuating diet." A fasting-based approach to epilepsy treatment was revived in the 1920s by the American osteopath and faith healer Hugh Conklin of Battle Creek, Michigan, who recommended an eighteen- to twenty-five-day "water diet."

Fasting was also used in ancient times to detoxify the body and purify the mind as a way to reach complete natural health. The Greek philosopher Pythagoras made his disciples do a forty-day fast before he would teach them his philosophy. He claimed that only after a fast of forty days would the minds of his followers be sufficiently purified and clarified to understand the profound teachings of life's mysteries. Even Benjamin Franklin gave us his opinion that "the best of all medicines is resting and fasting."

A 2014 peer-reviewed paper by Drs. Valter Longo and NIH researcher Mark Mattson, stated, "We now know that fasting results in ketogenesis; promotes potent changes in metabolic pathways and cellular processes such as stress resistance, lipolysis, and autophagy; and can have medical applications that, in some cases, are as effective as those of approved drugs such as the dampening of seizures and seizure-associated brain damage and the amelioration of rheumatoid arthritis."[17]

Mark Mattson, a neurosciences professor at Johns Hopkins School of Medicine and chief of the Laboratory of Neurosciences at the National Institute on Aging, is a prolific researcher in this area. He knows that fasting confers more than just benefits for people prone to seizures (much more coming in the next chapter on the history of epilepsy and ketogenic diets), and he has been involved in some of the studies I've already covered. He is particularly interested in how fasting can improve cognitive function and reduce the risk of developing neurodegenerative diseases. Dr. Mattson has conducted studies in which he subjected animals to alternative-day fasting, with a 10 to 25 percent calorie-restricted diet on the in-between days. According to him, "If you repeat that when animals are young, they live 30 percent longer."[18] The animals' nerve cells were more resistant to degeneration. And when he performed similar studies in women over the course of several weeks, he found that they lost more body fat, retained more lean muscle mass, and had an improvement in blood sugar control.[19]

Ironically, one of the mechanisms that triggers these biological reactions is not just autophagy but *stress*. During the fasting period, cells are under a mild stress, and they respond to that stress by enhancing their ability to cope with it and, maybe, to resist disease. Other studies have confirmed these findings.[20] When fasting is done correctly, it reduces blood pressure, improves insulin sensitivity, boosts kidney function, enhances brain function, regenerates the immune system, and increases resistance to diseases including cancer. The secret of leveraging fasting's power, however, lies in following a protocol that dials up autophagy while keeping your metabolism humming. In humans, depending upon their level of physical activity, a fast of twelve to twenty-four hours typically results in a 20 percent or greater decrease in blood sugar and depletion of the glycogen in the liver, thus triggering the burning of fat for energy.

You have probably already heard about intermittent fasting because various "fasting diets" have become popular. These programs (and the corresponding books) tout the ability to eat all you want if you limit yourself to one meal a day or suggest that you fast for two to three days a week and eat as much as you want on the remaining days. But here's the truth: there's no clear evidence that this will trigger the levels of autophagy that are required to improve one's health and lower the risk of disease. There are many ways to practice fasting, which I'll outline in chapter 9. The evidence to date says that the sweet spot is around sixteen hours, which you can easily do just by cutting yourself off from eating after 7:00 p.m. at night and skipping breakfast the next morning.[21] That's very doable. One common dietary theme, however, goes against conventional wisdom: we should be eating the bulk of our daily food *in the middle to early afternoon*.

If any single picture is beginning to come into plain view from studying dietary patterns among the longest-lived humans on the planet, it clearly does not involve three meals per day plus snacking, as per the typical American's grazing pattern. If you can fast overnight and skip breakfast a couple of times a week, as well as reduce your overall calorie consumption on some of the other days, you'll be well on your way to a healthier, stronger, more resilient you. At the very least, cut yourself off from eating a lot after a certain time, say 2:00 p.m. In fact, in 2019, Eric Ravussin of Pennington Biomedical Research Center took part in a study with the University of Alabama that led to a stunning paper showing the power of time-restricted eating on metabolism, markers of aging, and autophagy.[22] It was a small study involving only 11 people, but it nevertheless documented alarming results. When the subjects ate only between 8:00 a.m. and 2:00 p.m., as opposed to eating until 8:00 p.m., they experienced marked improvements in their twenty-four-hour glucose levels, signals of their circadian rhythm, and their expression of genes linked to aging and autophagy. (Note: All this timing talk may sound confusing, but you won't have to devise your own time-restricted plan; I'll be giving you a few options to follow.)

Another key dietary strategy that is often ignored is protein restriction. That's right: you don't want to be eating too much protein. Earlier I mentioned the power of protein turnover in the body, and protein restriction is related to this. Although the practice of general calorie restriction has benefits for body weight, it's really the protein restriction that creates the health benefits. If cutting way back on your calorie consumption sounds like a horrendous proposition and you don't need to lose weight, I've got good news for you: restriction of protein consumption—*without restricting calories*—is among the most promising interventions that have emerged to promote healthy aging in humans. And it's not going to feel as though you're "restricting" yourself, which is why it's better to call it *protein cycling*.

THE PERILS OF TOO MUCH PROTEIN

Protein is essential for the body to grow and repair itself. Protein-rich foods such as meat, eggs, fish, legumes, and dairy products get broken down into amino acids in the stomach and absorbed in the small intestine. The liver then sorts out which amino acids your body needs and the rest are flushed out in your urine. Protein provides the structural support of every cell in your body, and it's a component of skin, joints, bones, nails, muscles, and more. Without getting overly complicated, proteins are also involved in your immune system function, hormone regulation, and transmission of signals from one organ to another.

Adults who aren't especially active are advised to eat roughly 0.75 gram of protein per day for each kilogram they weigh. On average, this comes to 55 grams for men and 45 grams for women—or two palm-sized portions of meat, fish, tofu, or nuts. Not consuming enough protein can lead to loss of muscle strength and function, thinning hair, skin breakouts, and weight decline as muscle mass decreases. But these side effects are very rare and largely occur only in those with eating disorders. A more troubling common problem is consuming *too much protein.*

When one reads about so-called Blue Zones—areas around the world where genetics or lifestyle has imbued the inhabitants with superior health and longevity, such as the Okinawans and Greek monks—the one location referenced in the United States is Loma Linda (Spanish for "Beautiful Hill"), California, just east of downtown Los Angeles. In 2005, *National Geographic* magazine featured Loma Linda as one of three places in the world with the highest human longevity. Unlike smoggy LA, Loma Linda is sparsely populated, and about 9,000 of its 23,000 inhabitants are members of the Seventh-Day Adventist Church. The residents who follow the teachings of the Seventh-Day Adventist Church, which advocates living a healthy life free of gluttony and excess, live about ten years longer than do Americans in other towns and cities. Church members are encouraged to exercise and avoid harmful substances such as tobacco, alcohol, and mind-altering substances. A well-balanced vegetarian diet that avoids the consumption of meat coupled with an intake of legumes, whole grains, nuts, fruits, and vegetables, along with a source of vitamin B_{12}, such as eggs, yogurt, cheese, or a supplement, is recommended. In short, the Loma Lindans' diets are much, much lower in protein (especially animal protein) than that of the average American. (According to the top scientists working in this field, the majority of Americans consume about twice as much protein as they need to.) One of the trends driving this protein-centric health movement is the fascination with "paleo" or "caveman" and carnivore-type diets.

Due to the focus on restricting refined carbohydrates and sugar, the popular caveman-style diets have their merits. But these diets have a dark side: going low carb/paleo often results in eating too much of animal-derived proteins, which will work against you in many ways.[23] Among the surprising effects created by high-protein diets:

+ **Kidney damage:** Consuming lots of protein is hard on the kidneys, which have to filter out excess nitrogen found in the amino acids that make up the protein. This is especially problematic for anyone who has preexisting kidney disease or is vulnerable to such disease.

✦ **Weight gain:** Although weight loss is typical in the short term, eventually all that excess protein will be stored as fat, with surplus amino acids excreted in the urine.

✦ **Increased risk of developing heart disease:** A high-protein diet often includes more saturated fat and cholesterol, both of which are associated with an increased risk of developing cardiovascular disease. Moreover, a 2018 study showed that long-term consumption of red meat increases trimethylamine N-oxide (TMAO), a gut-generated chemical that is linked to heart disease.[24]

✦ **Increased cancer risk:** Many high-protein diets endorse the consumption of red meat–based protein. Multiple studies have shown that eating more red and processed meats is associated with certain kinds of cancer, particularly those of the breast, prostate, and colon. In fact, in a 2014 study that tracked a large sample of adults for nearly two decades, researchers found that eating a diet rich in animal proteins during middle age makes you four times more likely to die of cancer than someone following a low-protein diet—a mortality risk factor comparable to smoking.[25] The culprit here is the increased levels of growth hormone IGF-1 that accompany the protein intake. The research shows that for every 10 nanograms per milliliter (10 ng/ml) increase in IGF-1, those on a high-protein diet during middle age were 9 percent more likely to die from cancer than were those on a low-protein diet. That same 2014 study also revealed that people between the ages of 50 and 65 who are on a high-protein diet (defined as 20 percent or more of daily calories are coming from protein) had a 75 percent increase in overall mortality and a whopping 73 times greater risk of diabetes-related mortality. People in the moderate protein category (10 to 20 percent of calories from protein) had an almost 23-fold increase in the risk of diabetes mortality and a 3 times higher risk of cancer mortality than the low-protein group (less than 10 percent of calories from protein). Which brings me to the metabolic consequences . . .

✦ **Increased risk of developing metabolic disorders:** We often hear that too much sugar increases the risk of developing glucose intolerance, insulin resistance, and type 2 diabetes. But protein? Turns out it can dramatically raise your risks for these conditions as well. Studies going back to the mid-1990s show that high-protein diets are associated with glucose intolerance, insulin resistance, and an increased incidence of type 2 diabetes. A 2017 study in *The Journal of the American Medical Association* examined the deaths of more than 700,000 people in 2012 from heart disease, stroke, and type 2 diabetes.[26] They found that nearly 50 percent of the deaths were related to poor nutritional choices. For those who already had diabetes, the risk of death increased if they consumed more processed meats (in the past fifty years, there's been about a 33 percent rise in the consumption of processed meat). When researchers at the Harvard School of Public Health analyzed data from longitudinal studies of male and female health care professionals who were followed for fourteen to twenty-eight years, they calculated that a daily serving of red meat no bigger than a deck of cards increased the risk of adult-onset diabetes by 19 percent.[27] That was after adjusting for other risk factors. The worst villains were processed red meat such as hot dogs and bacon: a daily serving of processed red meat half that size was associated with a 51 percent increase in risk. (The average ten-year risk of getting diabetes for US adults is around 10 percent.) Another study released in 2017 by researchers in Finland analyzed the diets of more than 2,300 middle-aged men ages 42 to 60.[28] At the outset, none of the participants had type 2 diabetes. In the follow-up, after nineteen years, 432 of the participants did. Researchers found that those who consumed more animal protein and less plant protein had a 35 percent greater risk of getting diabetes. That included any kind of meat: both processed and unprocessed red meat, white meat, and variety meat, including organ meats such as tongue and liver.

I cannot emphasize the following enough: protein stimulates insulin release as much as carbohydrate does! We often don't think about that because we tend to relate insulin release with only sugar. One of insulin's jobs is to send amino acids from broken-down proteins into lean tissues such as muscle. But here's the difference: protein doesn't supply glucose rapidly, as carbohydrate does. If this process were to go unchecked, eating a high-protein meal would cause hypoglycemia (low blood sugar) because the release of insulin would suppress the blood glucose level too much. Glucagon release counterbalances insulin, preventing hypoglycemia when we eat a high-protein meal. However, certain amino acids that appear to be more potent in meat and dairy products than in vegetables, such as leucine and isoleucine, not only greatly stimulate insulin release but, unlike other amino acids, shut off rather than promote glucagon release. It's believed that these amino acids, as well as tryptophan, which increases insulin release much more than the other amino acids do, are largely responsible for the increase in obesity and insulin resistance that accompanies a chronic intake of high levels of meat and dairy products.

Where does health-promoting autophagy fit into this protein picture? Well, when you reduce your protein intake, especially animal proteins, you will lower your insulin levels and in turn boost your glucagon level and activate autophagy. This explains why protein cycling, or reducing your protein intake in cyclical fashion, has an effect similar to that of fasting. One of the main reasons protein cycling works to enhance youth is that your body can't create its own protein. Instead, it is forced to find every possible way to recycle the existing protein you've already provided it. Our bodies can handle periods without protein. If you think about it, this goes back to our ancestors, including the hunter-gatherers, who often had to survive for long stretches of time without a successful hunt. In addition to enhancing autophagy, protein cycling alongside calorie restriction and intermittent fasting will help reduce your risk of developing the diseases I've covered: diabetes, cancer, and heart disease. Remember, these are the diseases of civilization, also known as diseases of overconsumption.

Protein cycling could become your most powerful tool for making over your metabolism and increasing your chances of living a long, disease-free life. This is especially helpful for people who find it unrealistic to commit to the rigors of calorie restriction and fasting. I will offer several different strategies in chapter 9 that you can tailor to your own preferences. For some people, a rhythmic mix of CR, fasting, and protein cycling will work and be practical. Others will need a less demanding protocol. I get it; we're all different and have our own individual health challenges, goals, risk factors, and lifestyle choices. The key for you will be establishing a baseline framework to follow throughout much of the year, building in the habits that you find doable and effective—and that help you meet your goals.

Finally, I should say a little more about dairy products.

SPILLING THE MILK

The documented effects of dairy products on the body (and their dampening of autophagy) are so compelling that I will caution that, in my opinion, we shouldn't be regularly consuming dairy products made from cow's milk in high quantities as grown adults. Early hominins, like all other mammals, would have drunk the milk of their own species during the nursing period. After weaning, however, the consumption of milk and milk products of other mammals would have been nearly impossible before the domestication of livestock. Imagine the task of capturing and milking wild mammals. Although sheep were domesticated by 9,000 BCE, and goats and cows by 8,000 BCE, historical evidence for dairying dates to 4100–3500 BCE in the form of residues of dairy fats found on pottery in Great Britain. These clues show that dairy foods are relative newcomers to the hominin diet, at least on an evolutionary timescale.

The phrase "Finish your milk" is familiar to most of us who grew up under the influence of the famous "Got milk?" and "Milk mustache" campaigns of the 1980s and '90s. The ubiquitous ads implored us to drink milk daily if we wanted to grow up healthy and strong (and be like our favorite athletes and celebrities). Drinking milk when you're growing and developing is one thing, but consuming lots of dairy as an adult is another. Since the original milk campaigns, milk's health halo has been tainted by concerns about its potential role in the rising rates of obesity, diabetes, allergies, digestive disorders, and other chronic health problems. Case-control (observational) studies in diverse populations have shown a strong and consistent association between serum IGF-1 concentrations and prostate cancer risk.[29] Increased IGF-1 has been shown in lab studies to promote the growth of cancerous prostate cells.

Another issue with dairy products is the process of pasteurization. Though this process does reduce the small risk of milk contamination, it kills off the beneficial bacteria (probiotics) in the milk, alters milk proteins from their natural state, and transforms milk from a source of nutrition into a source of potential health problems in some people. Pasteurization also converts milk's lactose sugars into beta-lactose sugars that the body absorbs faster, causing blood sugar spikes.

Lots of people have trouble digesting cow's milk due to its whey and casein proteins. Consumption of whey increases the body's insulin level (which can lead to insulin resistance and a high blood glucose level and in turn inflammation), and casein promotes the release of IGF-1 (which keeps mTOR activated and autophagy off, as previously noted). Casein has also been shown to trigger an immune response in some people, which will, of course, raise the body's level of inflammation.[30] One of the reasons many body builders develop acne is partly due to their consumption of whey-based protein shakes and bars (and the synthetic steroids that some use don't help either). Both whey and casein have long been implicated in the development of acne. During the program, I'll ask that you try to shift away from cow's milk and turn to non-animal-protein-based alternatives such as almond, flax, or hemp milk. For those of you who truly want a traditional milk, sheep's milk can be a possibility. People who develop an intolerance to cow's (and even goat's) milk often find that sheep's milk products, including certain cheeses, are the only dairy products they can safely eat.

If I had to say which dietary pattern is the most problematic, I'd call out the overconsumption of both dairy products and animal protein. You might think I'd name sugar and bad fats and salt, but when you think about it, a lot of excess sugar, fat, and salt ride along with meals heavy in processed animal proteins and dairy products (just think of the classic American fare of a cheeseburger with fries and a milkshake). What you often don't hear about is the fact that dairy products and meat contain a large amount of three amino acids in particular that will shut down autophagy. They are called leucine, isoleucine, and valine and are what's known in nutrition circles as branched-chain amino acids (BCAAs) due to their molecular structure. Although we need these essential amino acids in our diets to carry out certain functions in the body, most people consume way too much of them, with far-reaching implications for their health. It's well documented that lowering the intake of BCAAs from animal sources can improve metabolism, but newer research has shown that they can even impact hormones and estrogen receptors.

In 2019, for example, it was reported in the journal *Nature* that women being treated for breast cancer can lose their response to a chemotherapy drug such as tamoxifen if their diets are high in leucine.[31] Leucine turns on mTOR, which increases cell division and proliferation. Leucine increases the proliferation not only of normal cells but also of breast cancer cells, while decreasing leucine levels suppresses it. Put another way, you can turn down cell proliferation and starve a cancer by limiting your intake of leucine. Indeed, diet can be anticancerous. I think this speaks volumes for the 1 in 8 women who will develop breast cancer in her life. Most of these cancers (fully 75 percent), are made up of estrogen receptor–positive cells that need estrogen and/or progesterone to grow. In general, the reason people who consume a lot of body-building protein shakes and bars have a higher risk of developing cancer is the presence of BCAAs in the supplemental proteins they are taking.

BCAAs do serve a purpose in the body and are required for growth and repair, but we'd do well to consume them in moderation, largely from plant sources. And when you're focusing on dialing up autophagy for certain months of the year, you'll want to avoid these nutrients. Again, if you follow the dietary protocol outlined in chapter 9, you'll automatically be reducing your intake when you should without having to pay much attention to how to do it.

CHAPTER 5

EPILEPTIC CHILDREN AND WORLD-CLASS CYCLISTS

In ancient Greece, epilepsy was known as the "falling-down illness." Way back then, nobody knew what triggered episodes of a person suddenly twitching, convulsing, showing signs of paralysis, and perhaps foaming at the mouth. Before the Greeks, the Babylonians believed that demons and ghosts, which they thought could possess a person temporarily, caused illnesses such as epilepsy. (In the ancient Babylonian language, the verb meaning "to seize" also carries a meaning "to possess," and that word was applied to epilepsy.) Of course, we now know that supernatural spells have nothing to do with epilepsy. The condition is caused by a disruption of nerve cell activity in the brain that causes seizures, often unpredictably. During a seizure, the person experiences unusual behavior such as uncontrolled jerking movements, an abnormal sensation or feeling of movement called an aura, and sometimes a loss of awareness or consciousness—hence the "falling-down" description. It's the fourth most common neurological disorder and affects people of all ages. Some people are born with the condition, while others develop it over time; children affected by epilepsy may outgrow it with age, though for many it's a lifelong condition.

Although there are different types of seizures, with multiple circumstances causing epilepsy—from genetics and developmental disorders to head trauma, brain conditions, and infectious diseases—luckily we have effective ways of treating it today through medication, dietary interventions, and, if appropriate, surgery. Dietary therapy has a long history, and for thousands of years it was the only method doctors had to treat an epileptic brain. It remains one of the most potent, drug-free ways to manage this condition, which is largely only controlled, not cured. How we came to identify the link between diet and brain function, especially with regard to epilepsy, highlights the power of observation. It was during periods as far back as ancient Greece that prescient physicians took note of what happened when food supplies ran low. Leave it to the Greeks to look past notions of paranormal causes of illness; they introduced the concept of natural causation of disease, though it would take thousands of years to truly understand the causes of epilepsy.

Before the development of modern farming and food distribution industries, humans went through frequent and sometimes devastatingly severe famines throughout history. Since the fifth century BCE, Greek physicians, observing the effects of mild famine on epileptics, recommended fasting or periodic starvation to treat the illness (not calling in an exorcist, as the Babylonians had done). In the early 1900s, physicians in France and the United

States once again pointed to fasting to treat epilepsy. Sometime around 1920, doctors noticed that patients undergoing starvation or fasting had acetone on their breath and beta-hydroxybutyric acid in their blood. Dr. Russell Wilder, an endocrinologist at the Mayo Clinic in Rochester, Minnesota, decided that this was caused by ketogenesis, the production of ketones from fatty acids. Acetone and beta-hydroxybutyric acid are two of the three ketone compounds that occur naturally throughout the body under certain conditions. Those conditions include carbohydrate restriction, as when intentionally fasting or undergoing starvation during a famine. Ketones are water-soluble molecules made in the liver. Because prolonged starving isn't healthy for children (among other things, it stunts their growth and development), Dr. Wilder proposed attempting to treat epileptic children by putting them on a high-fat, low-carbohydrate diet that he called the "ketogenic diet." He suggested that this diet could be as effective in mediating their epilepsy symptoms as fasting and could be maintained for a much longer period of time.

Dr. Wilder is now credited with originally designing the ketogenic diet. He was a pioneer in medicine in a lot of ways, in fact. A long-established expert in metabolism and nutrition, he devoted much of his career to type 1 diabetes patients, most of whom were children. He was a leader in the clinical use of insulin soon after its discovery by a couple of Canadian doctors at the University of Toronto (before then, type 1 diabetics often didn't live long once the condition developed). Dr. Wilder played an instrumental role in determining proper insulin dosing. In 1931, he became head of the department of medicine at the Mayo Clinic and was a staunch advocate for more research in nutrition. He also played an important part in the development of the American Diabetes Association and served as its president in 1947, close to his retirement.

In the 1960s, Dr. Peter Huttenlocher of the University of Chicago substituted a class of saturated fats called medium-chain triglycerides (MCTs) for other forms of oil in the diet, because MCTs produce more ketones and thereby allowed dieters to consume more carbohydrates than were allowed under the standard keto diet. (The majority of fat in most Western diets is made up of long-chain fatty acids, which contain 13 to 21 carbons. In contrast, the medium-chain fatty acids in MCTs have 6 to 12 carbon atoms. You may have heard of "MCT oil," which is documented to improve cognitive function and weight management. Coconut oil is a good source of MCTs and the reason behind coconut oil's health claims.) By 1970, Dr. Samuel Livingston of Johns Hopkins Hospital in Baltimore, was writing about the results of more than 1,000 epileptic children who had followed a ketogenic diet. Of them, more than 50 percent had complete control of their seizures while on the diet, and another 27 percent had improved control. However, as antiseizure drugs, such as Dilantin (phenytoin) and sodium valproate, began being marketed to doctors for the treatment of epilepsy, the ketogenic diet lost favor, and it was not revived until 1994, largely through the efforts of a Hollywood producer, Jim Abrahams, who desperately began searching for a cure for his son's devastating epileptic seizures. He eventually met Dr. John Freeman, a 60-year-old pediatric neurologist who worked with epileptic children at Johns Hopkins School of Medicine. Dr. Freeman was challenging the medical establishment by advocating the revival of the ketogenic diet as a drug-free, side effect–free treatment for intractable epilepsy. Within two days of his starting the ketogenic diet, Jim's son's seizures vanished. A *Dateline NBC* episode that covered this story in 1994 reignited the case for the ketogenic diet, and today such a diet is considered a mainstream medical treatment in addition to other therapies, and is prescribed in more than forty-five countries. The combination of antiepileptic drugs and the ketogenic diet can help many people successfully control their seizures.

For a long time we didn't understand the mechanism behind the diet's effects on an epileptic brain, but after a seminal study out of Emory University Health Sciences in 2005, it's been thought that the diet alters the genes involved in energy metabolism in the brain, which in turn helps stabilize the function of neurons exposed to the challenges of epileptic seizures.[1] Newer studies indicate that the diet may be an effective additional treatment for autism, brain tumors (glioblastoma in particular), polycystic ovarian syndrome, obesity and other metabolic syndromes, acne, amyotrophic lateral sclerosis (ALS, also known as Lou Gehrig's disease), Alzheimer's disease, Parkinson's disease, diabetes, mood disorders, and major depression. In mice, the diet improves hippocampal memory deficits and extends healthy life span.[2] So it has multiple effects on the body from the brain on down.

At the heart of the ketogenic diet is its super-low-carb content, high fat intake (typically 70 to 80 percent of calories come from fat), and moderate protein intake. This raises the question: Does the body really need carbohydrates for basic functioning? We are often told that glucose is the body's main and preferred source of fuel, especially for the brain. We are also told to limit our consumption of fat intake to 20 percent of total calories a day. What do the data show?

ENDURANCE ATHLETES REVEAL THE SECRETS

The data that began to reveal the complete opposite—that the body can perform its best on virtually zero carbs and mostly fat—dates as far back as 1983, when Stephen Phinney published a study with his colleagues at MIT and Harvard on world-class competitive cyclists who went on a ketogenic diet for four weeks.[3] Some of the participants *increased* their endurance, which was an unexpected outcome given the conventional wisdom. The diet consisted of 15 percent of calories from protein, 83 percent from fat, and less than 3 percent (fewer than 20 grams) of carbohydrate daily (the equivalent of one potato, half a hamburger bun, or a small serving of pasta). They underwent VO2 max (measuring maximal oxygen uptake) and endurance tests before and after the diet. It was a very small study that had its hiccups (one of the subjects had reduced performance after the diet, but he was found to be overtrained, which skewed the results; when his results were excluded, the average boost in endurance was 13 percent). The study nonetheless marked the beginning of a new era in diet mentality that would unfold with future investigations. At the time, Phinney's work went mostly unnoticed because he was called a "heretic" in the field, but he later went on to become a professor emeritus at UC Davis and continued to publish these kinds of findings among endurance athletes as recently as 2018.[4]

Nobody in the 1980s, however, wanted to take seriously a high-fat diet as a way to lose weight, achieve peak performance, and perhaps even prevent heart disease. It just didn't seem to make sense, given the thinking at the time: Eat fat to lose fat? Eat fat to get faster? Eat fat to avoid heart disease? But times have changed. Today we have plenty of evidence to show the value of ketogenic diets, including studies with Dr. Phinney and others around the world.[5] And the benefits are not only for endurance athletes or people with epilepsy. Dr. Phinney now works primarily with people seeking sustained weight loss and better management of metabolic conditions, chiefly diabetes. He cofounded a company that helps people with prediabetes and diabetes reverse their conditions largely through diet, consuming a low-carb, high-fat diet, or what he has coined "nutritional ketosis." In as little as ten weeks, some of his patients cure their diabetes and no longer need insulin. It's staggering when you think about it: if an eating plan can alleviate a disease as serious as diabetes in a matter of weeks, imagine what it can do for a body that's not saddled with a metabolic condition to start with!

THE SCIENCE OF THE KETOGENIC DIET

The ketogenic diet is similar to fasting in many metabolic and physiological respects, which is one of the reasons I started reading research papers about it and self-experimenting with the diet in 2013. Ultimately, I followed a vegan ketogenic diet myself for more than three years (more about that later). My question was: Could the diet be used to mimic the mTOR-suppressing and autophagy-inducing results of fasting while still including substantial calories? The good news is that it likely can, if implemented properly. The bad news is that, unlike calorie restriction, fasting, and protein restriction, we can't really point to any culture or "health oasis" groups (such as Laron syndrome dwarfs, Okinawan centenarians, Loma Linda vegans, or Mount Athos monks) who have saved us the trouble of running clinical trials to show us the long-term antiaging health benefits. Instead, we're going to have to delve into the science of how the ketogenic diet works and why it *should* mimic the beneficial results of those other mTOR/autophagy-switching lifestyles.

The Keto Math

At any given time, the average 150-pound individual has about 80 calories of glucose (the equivalent of six to seven sugar cubes) coursing through 5 liters of blood. Glucose that's stored in the muscles (called glycogen) is equal to about 480 calories, and stored in the liver are another 280 calories of glycogen, for a total of about 880 calories ready for use. To get a perspective, that same 150-pound person would burn about 46 calories an hour sleeping, 68 an hour sitting quietly, 102 per hour doing light work such as shopping or general milling about, and 170 per hour doing moderate work such as household chores or gardening. If the last meal were eaten at 6:00 p.m., followed by four hours of sitting and then eight hours of sleep, the individual would use up roughly three-fourths of his or her stored glucose/glycogen (stored energy) by 6:00 a.m. (Note: I realize that this math pertains only to a 150-pound individual and that the numbers differ depending on weight, height, age, and gender. The published research upon which these calculations are based typically refers to an "average 150-pound *man*." Most American men today who are a tad above 5 feet, 9 inches tall weigh at least 20 pounds more than that. But for purposes of this explanation, let's use the 150-pound reference point. The overall lesson remains the same.)

Whenever you substantially limit your carbohydrate intake for longer than twelve hours, you're likely to burn through that tiny amount of stored glucose and glycogen in your body and cause your body to turn to its "real" source of stored energy—fat. A 150-pound man with a body composition of 22 percent fat would have 33 pounds of adipose-tissue triglycerides, amounting to 135,000 calories, available for use. (This percentage would be considered "overweight" for men, but it's still far below that of the obese, who have more than 25 percent body fat and who currently include about 50 percent of Americans over 65.) At several thousand calories of daily expenditure, you can see that that fat would get him through several months of nonstop fasting or famine.

When the body burns through stored glucose and glycogen and starts burning fat, the liver produces the alternative fuel I mentioned called ketone bodies. You are "in ketosis" when ketone bodies accumulate in the blood. All of us experience mild ketosis when we fast, when we get up the morning after a long, glucose-deprived sleep, or after very strenuous exercise. Ketosis has been an important adaptation throughout human evolution, allowing us to persevere when adequate food was hard to find. According to science journalist Gary Taubes, the author of *Why We Get Fat: And What to Do About It*, "In fact, we can define this mild ketosis as the normal state of human metabolism when we're not eating the carbohydrates that didn't exist in our diets for 99.9 percent of human history. As such, ketosis is arguably not just a natural condition but even a particularly healthful one."[6]

Throughout our evolution, we sought fat (especially fatty organs such as liver, brains, and bone marrow) as a calorie-dense food source. It's likely one of the reasons large animals (mammoths, woolly rhinos, and giant sloths) all disappeared from northern regions as the human population there was expanding: those animals were great sources of fat in addition to protein. We should also remember that many of our ancestors suffered through a 20,000-year-long mini–ice age, in which the supply of carbohydrates would have been limited to a few short summer months of the year (as they are even now in Arctic Circle areas, such as Alaska and northern Canada). This may also be the reason why humans developed such a taste for sweet things and especially carbohydrates; it was nature's way of making sure we'd take as much advantage of their limited availability as possible. For the rest of the year, however, fat was what kept us healthy, lean, and energized during our hunter-gatherer days.

As you already know, eating carbohydrates stimulates insulin production. Consumption of too many carbs and the resulting production of insulin are what lead to fat production and fat storage. And, as you can imagine, such a scenario means a reduced ability to burn fat. Manufacturers of processed foods continue to put the term "low-fat" on their labels to enhance sales of what are mostly high-glycemic processed foods. And that's where the problem starts, with products that will dramatically increase your blood glucose levels, increase your appetite, release insulin that tells your body to make more fat and "spare" burning the fat you already have, and keep autophagy turned down as low as possible because your metabolic switch is constantly turned to the growth cycle. Studies done more than twenty years ago have documented higher mortality rates among people with high carb consumption and lower mortality rates (and lower risk of developing cardiovascular disease) among people with higher fat consumption. More recently, in a 2017 study published in the highly regarded journal *The Lancet*, researchers from multiple esteemed institutions around the world analyzed more than 135,000 individuals aged 35 to 70 years from eighteen countries over an average of 7.4 years.[7] They grouped them according to the amount of carbohydrates, fat, and protein they consumed, using self-reported dietary data from the participants. Further, they compared the diets to the risk of developing various conditions, including a major cardiovascular event, stroke, heart failure, and death.

What the researchers discovered went against the conventional wisdom: when they compared the highest consumers of carbohydrates (77 percent of daily calories) with the lowest (46 percent of daily calories), higher carbohydrate consumption was associated with a 28 percent increased risk of death. Conversely, the researchers found that those with the highest intake of dietary fat (35 percent of daily calories) were 23 percent less likely to have died than those with the lowest intake of fat (10 percent of daily calories). The study tried to tease out different types of fats and their effects, finding that those who consumed the highest levels of polyunsaturated and monounsaturated fats (e.g., the good fats found in many plant-based oils, nuts, seeds, avocados, and fish) experienced a 20 and 19 percent reduced risk of death, respectively. Even people who ate high levels of the "dreaded" saturated fat found in butter and animal meats had a 14 percent reduced risk of death.

The study did have its shortcomings because it grouped different types of carbohydrates together (carbs from vegetables are not the same as carbs from refined grains) and because relying on people's food dairies can be imprecise science. But the study nevertheless met the authors' goals of trying to move the spotlight from promoting low-fat diets to promoting a reduction in carbohydrate intake. More often than not, it's the refined carb-based diets that are killing us. The authors concluded, "High carbohydrate intake was associated with higher risk of total mortality, whereas total fat and individual types of fat were related to lower total mortality. Total fat and types of fat were not associated with cardiovascular disease, myocardial infarction, or cardiovascular disease mortality, whereas saturated fat had an inverse association with stroke. Global dietary guidelines should be reconsidered in light of these findings." That last statement is key; if only we could see more action taking place to change the dietary rule books around the world.

High-glycemic processed carbohydrates—not dietary fats—are the chief cause of weight gain. (And when you think about it, what do most farmers use to fatten their animals destined for the butcher block? High-glycemic carbohydrates such as corn and grain, rather than the low-glycemic, high-fiber grass and hay they evolved to eat.) This partly explains why weight loss—sometimes dramatic—is one of the major health effects of a low-carbohydrate diet. When your diet is continuously high in low-quality carbohydrates, which in effect keep your insulin pump on, you prevent the breakdown of your body fat for fuel. Your body becomes hooked on that glucose. You may even burn through your glucose but still not be able to access your fat for fuel due to the volume of insulin present in your body. The body essentially becomes physically starved, which is why many obese individuals struggle to lose weight while they continue to eat carbs. Their insulin levels lock the gate to those fat stores. Until they exchange their processed high-glycemic carbs for healthy fats, they will continue to swim in too much insulin and likely become diabetic if they are not already. In fact, switching to a keto-friendly whole-food diet is increasingly becoming the preferred method of treating type 2 diabetes. Stephen Phinney was onto this idea decades ago, but it's finally gaining acceptance now that the science has spoken loudly.

You may not be insulin resistant or diabetic. But by having an understanding of how the ketogenic diet can reverse serious metabolic conditions such as these will help you appreciate ketogenesis' powerful effects on physiology to spur fat burning and weight loss and, when used correctly, turn up autophagy. Being diabetic means the body is at a disadvantage because its metabolism is not working normally. It's sputtering like a machine that is not able to run efficiently due to glitches in its system and damaged parts. Enter the ketogenic diet, which acts like a tune-up to fix the damage and clean the engine. It can then run like new.

Dr. Sarah Hallberg is the medical director at Virta Health in California, where she collaborates with Dr. Phinney. She is also the founder and medical director of the Arnett Physicians Weight Loss Program at Indiana University. Dr. Hallberg and her colleagues conducted a study on a group of 349 type 2 diabetics.[8] Part of the group received standard care under the direction of their physicians over a one-year period; the other group was placed on a ketogenic diet. They started out at 30 grams of carbohydrates each day, and the level of carbohydrates was adjusted to keep them in ketosis. What was unique about the study was the fact that the intervention group—the one put on the ketogenic diet—was in close touch with health coaches and physicians, with frequent measurements of their blood sugar and hemoglobin A1c levels (a measurement of average blood glucose levels over the past three months), as well as their blood ketone level, to ensure that they maintained ketosis. In addition, their body weight and medication use were documented.

After one year, the patients on the ketogenic diet had lost 12 percent of their body weight and their glycated hemoglobin A1c level had gone down, a sign of improved blood glucose level. Briefly, glycation is the biochemical term for the bonding of sugar molecules to proteins, fats, and amino acids. Hemoglobin is the protein found in red blood cells that carries oxygen, and when it's exposed to glucose in the blood, they become bound together through the glycation process. This is why your glycated hemoglobin level is also a measure of your blood sugar level; your doctor likely measures your level during a routine physical exam. (It gives an average for the previous three months because that's the average life span of a red blood cell.) Fully 94 percent of patients who had previously been prescribed insulin were able to reduce or stop their insulin altogether. And the patients who were taking sulfonylureas, a common oral diabetic medication, were all able to discontinue the drug. The patients who did not go on the ketogenic diet had no changes in their hemoglobin A1c level, their weight, or their use of diabetes medication. It's important to reiterate that the group on the ketogenic diet was continuously supervised by a health coach and a doctor, and that also may have factored into their dramatic improvement, as they were less likely to cheat on or veer from the dietary protocol. This study, published in 2018, demonstrated that a ketogenic diet can be one of the most effective interventions for the treatment of type 2 diabetes.

A hemoglobin A1c level less than 5 percent and a blood glucose level of 75 to 90 milligrams per deciliter (mg/dL), independent of other factors, generally means healthier veins and eyes and a far lower risk of developing cardiovascular disease, cancer, and Alzheimer's disease.

How are ketones so helpful biologically? The answer, which is relevant for all of us whether we struggle with metabolic challenges or not, is that they produce beneficial biological changes. They make over our metabolism, or, as one prominent researcher likes to say, when we're in ketosis, we are "essentially reorganizing all of [our] metabolism."[9] In doing so, we decrease our blood sugar level and improve our insulin sensitivity, lower our level of inflammation, boost our production of antioxidants, and even increase our activation of the sirtuin gene, associated with increased life span in animals. Ketones also have the effect of eliminating our sugar cravings and hunger in general; we feel satisfied at every meal and don't need to count calories because the diet is self-limiting. It's hard to binge on avocados, leafy greens, and plant-based proteins.

In addition to the diet's being studied for having significant effects on metabolism and rescuing diabetics from a lifetime of drug dependence, numerous studies are currently under way to look into how it affects other systems, the central nervous system being one of them. This is not too surprising when you consider the fact that the health of one's general metabolism factors into the health of every system in the body. Even the brain's metabolism hinges on the main body's metabolism. This may help explain why, for example, a small pilot study in 2017 reported that Alzheimer's disease patients who followed the University of Kansas's ketogenic diet program for three months improved by an average of 4 points on one of the most important cognitive assessments in dementia care, the Alzheimer's Disease Assessment Scale–cognitive subscale (ADAS-cog).[10] The diet comprised 70 percent fat. In the words of Dr. Russell Swerdlow, who led the study and presented it at the Alzheimer's Association International Conference, "This is the most robust improvement in the ADAS-cog scale that I am aware of for an Alzheimer's interventional trial."[11] Rightly so, he's calling for more studies with many more participants to replicate such findings. Alzheimer's disease is increasingly being called "type 3 diabetes" because the disease does involve a disrupted relationship with insulin, and people with type 2 diabetes are at least twice as likely to develop the disease as those without. In a much larger study published earlier in 2015, a randomized clinical trial in an older population over the course of five years showed that a Mediterranean diet supplemented with olive oil or nuts (which are rich in poly- and monounsaturated fatty acids) is associated with improved cognitive function.[12]

Also in 2017 came two independent mouse studies—one led by a team at UC Davis and another by a team at the Buck Institute for Research on Aging—providing evidence that a ketogenic diet improves memory in older animals, as well as the chances that an animal will live a long life. The findings, published in the journal *Cell Metabolism*, offer clues that ketogenic diets can be used to improve both longevity and health span, or the period during which a person enjoys good health.[13] Mice in both studies were fed one of three diets starting in midlife: a regular rodent high-carb diet (essentially the control), a low-carb/high-fat diet, and a strict ketogenic diet with zero carbohydrate intake. Because the researchers initially worried that the high-fat diet would increase the rodents' weight and decrease their life span, they kept the calorie count of each diet the same. The purpose of the study was to focus on metabolism and aging—not weight loss per se. They tested their mice at various ages on tasks such as navigating mazes, staying aloft on balance beams, and running on wheels. More testing checked for heart function and gene regulation changes through RNA-sequencing analysis, which showed that the diets created insulin-signaling and gene-expression patterns typically found in fasting (no surprise there).

Though both studies showed improvements in midlife life span, memory tests, and age-related markers of inflammation, one of the studies also found that a ketogenic diet preserved physical fitness in old age.[14] (As an interesting aside, one of the ways physical fitness is measured in the context of aging is through grip strength and walking speed. Indeed, how strong you can make a fist and how fast you can walk are remarkable signs of how fast you are aging.) Previous studies have also found that one ketone body in particular, beta-hydroxybutyrate, produced by the diet not only functions as fuel but also produces cell signaling.[15] Beta-hydroxybutyrate cell signaling might help make an animal resistant to oxidative stress, which is one of the pathways of aging.

Ketosis and Autophagy

If following a ketogenic diet is similar physiologically to calorie restriction and fasting, you'd assume that it triggers autophagy. Indeed, ketosis can be a gateway to autophagy. But you can be in ketosis without autophagy, and you can have autophagy without being in ketosis. The two don't always go hand in hand (i.e., being tested for ketones in your body will not mean that you're also being tested to see if autophagy is on). Whether you're in one state or the other—or in both at the same time—depends on what you eat and when. Recall that autophagy is activated during energy deprivation, which can be the result of reducing your intake of glucose and proteins, fasting, and exercise. Your metabolism needs low insulin, low mTOR, and high AMPK levels for autophagy to be turned on. The depletion of glycogen in the liver and carbohydrate deficiencies is what leads to the creation of ketone bodies. Without glucose available for fuel, the body jump-starts the ketone-manufacturing process using fat. What this means is that you can consume foods that will keep you in ketosis but will halt autophagy. By the same token, autophagy doesn't require ketosis to be activated; you can have autophagy dialed up without being in ketosis. Again, it all boils down to what you eat: the composition of your food, your calorie intake, and whether or not you're intermittently fasting.

Generally speaking, being in ketosis already meets a lot of the prerequisites of autophagy, including low insulin, low blood glucose, and lower mTOR levels. If you're not consuming too many carbs or too much protein on a daily basis, you can expect to go into autophagy faster than someone who first has to burn through all of his or her stored glucose. Since your body gets good at switching into burning fat mode for its energy, you'll also be far less hungry when you miss a meal or go on a multiday fast. The most natural and effective way of simultaneously activating autophagy *and* ketosis is to fast for several days, an option I will give you when I outline program protocols. This causes energy depletion and ramps up ketone production. Aside from fasting, a therapeutic ketogenic diet that incorporates some form of intermittent fasting (not more than two meals a day) is the closest you can get to an autophagy-mimicking diet. To turn on autophagy while on a ketogenic diet, you just have to make sure you're not eating too frequently, you're practicing some form of time-restricted eating, you're not eating too much protein, and you stay physically active. However, those same principles also apply to other diets such as vegan, carnivore, and paleo. I will help you figure this all out during the program so you can choose to balance the benefits of turning autophagy on and trying a ketogenic diet. You'll ideally want to be in both states at various times throughout the year.

The ketogenic diet is not for everyone, and it's not to be followed every day of the year. I go on it sporadically throughout the year at specified intervals and include intermittent fasting and calorie restriction to accelerate autophagy. But there actually is a time when ketogenic diets should be suspended. Unfortunately, most keto diet proponents do not cover this important ground. In 2018, the ketogenic diet was listed low on the list of "best diets" endorsed by doctors and dieticians. The reason, however, is that many people go about the diet wrong and think that it allows them to snack on bacon and other processed meats daily or eat as much saturated fat as their heart desires. Because ketogenic diets favor fat in the diet, you need to be careful about which kind of fat you take in (more unsaturated fats from olive oil, avocados, and certain nuts; less bad fats from cheese, butter, dairy products, and meat). Going keto will be an option to try in the program outlined in chapter 9. I will provide general dietary guidelines that we all should be following with an option to go keto.

I should add that there's often a transition period for entering ketosis, and it can take several days once you start the ketogenic diet. During this time, you may experience fatigue, light-headedness, "brain fog," headaches, irritability, muscle cramps, and nausea. This is to be expected as part of your metabolism makeover. A lot of these negative effects are due to the loss of fluid and electrolytes such as sodium—both of which are held by the carbs. When you drastically cut back on your carb consumption, you no longer have those vehicles for water and electrolytes. There are ways to mediate this, however, with certain supplements, notably the B vitamins. After the transition, you're said to be "keto adapted," meaning your body has gone through the transition of relying mostly on glucose for fuel to relying mostly on fat. About a week to ten days into a ketogenic diet, you will start to feel better with increased energy, stamina, and vitality. The body continues to make additional subtle changes over the course of several more weeks. For example, it gradually becomes more conserving of protein, so you'll often crave less protein. Another change that athletes in particular often notice is less fatigue and soreness due to less lactic acid buildup in their muscles after long training sessions.

You can determine if you're in ketosis by measuring the ketones in your urine using over-the-counter meters and test strips you can find at a local pharmacy. The effective therapeutic range of ketone levels in an individual's blood is 0.5 to 4.0 millimolar (mM), but maintaining this long term can be a challenge. There's also a "breaking in" period during which many people who go on the diet feel bad before feeling better, suffering from what's often called "keto flu." This is normal and simply a response to the body's shifting gears from using glucose to using fat for fuel. Once your body is "keto adapted," however, it becomes easier to shift into and out of the diet without these symptoms.

In chapter 9, I will suggest a standard keto diet for those who want to accelerate their results. The tricky part of this diet is ensuring that you're reducing your carb intake enough while not becoming deficient in certain nutrients, fiber, minerals, and vitamins or sacrificing lean body mass. For this reason, and as I mentioned before, some people would do well to take supplements while on the diet. Everyone's carb intake to stay in ketosis will be different: some people will need to eat fewer carbs to stay in ketosis; those who are heavy exercisers can get away with more, as their muscles will be burning through the glucose. Other factors, such as stress and hormones, can also come into play.

All people come to the proverbial table with a different set of risk factors. I, for example, inherited several genetic variants that link high total cholesterol and LDL cholesterol (the so-called bad cholesterol) levels to saturated dietary fat intake. One month on coconut oil (which is high in saturated fat) made my total cholesterol level double and substantially raised my bad cholesterol level. Since ketogenesis is brought about by limiting your carbohydrate level until your cells switch to burning fat, it doesn't matter what type of dietary fat you choose to substitute for those calories. But you should choose wisely so you don't bring on other health conditions. In my case, I quickly got off the coconut oil and decided to substitute some polyunsaturated fatty acids and a lot more monounsaturated fatty acids (discussed in depth in chapter 7) for the missing calories. Within a month my total cholesterol levels had not only returned to my preketo levels but had reduced by another 50 percent (the best I'd ever seen).

Although the ketogenic diet is a trend (and term) that has gained popularity only in the last decade or so, thanks in part to the science finally catching up to all the anecdotal evidence for its biological benefits, I'd bet that our long-lost (lean, energetic, athletic) ancestors from eons ago roamed the planet in ketosis much of the year. They had to because high-carb meals were not down the street (or behind the next tree). Sugary junk food didn't exist. And there were no grocery stores filled with refined carbohydrate-laden cereals, baked goods, snacks, and high-fructose corn syrup–rich soft drinks. They ate the way we should today.

CHAPTER 6

CAVEMEN AND INDUSTRIALISTS

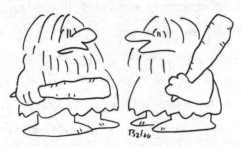

"I'm tired of hunting and gathering, too, but nobody's *invented* grocery stores yet."

CartoonStock.com

In 1956, Dr. James Neel founded the nation's first academic department of human genetics at the University of Michigan, just a few years after DNA's twisted-ladder molecular structure was decoded. Dr. Neel was a pioneer in human genetics—the first scientist to recognize the genetic basis for sickle cell anemia, which led to the rare disorder becoming the first described "molecular disease" (like Laron syndrome, sickle cell anemia is inherited in an autosomal recessive pattern, which means that mutations must be inherited from both parents; having only one copy makes a person a carrier).

Although Neel is probably best known for his extensive studies of Hiroshima and Nagasaki atomic bomb survivors and the effects of radiation on them and their offspring for more than forty years, it was his "thrifty gene" theory in the field of genetics and his studies of hunter-gatherer tribes in Brazil and Venezuela that stirred a revolution in scientific thinking. As proposed by Dr. Neel in 1962 and further elucidated in his 1998 follow-up article, the "thrifty genome," a genetic predisposition to quickly send glucose from our bloodstream into cells to be burned as fuel and stored as fat, would have given an evolutionary advantage to our tribal, hunter-gatherer ancestors. Inherited genes that massively increase the risk of developing (and predispose someone to) such diseases as diabetes, obesity, and high blood pressure stem from our early ancestors' need to store enough energy to survive long-lasting famines, yet have enough energy to outrun a saber-toothed tiger.[1] These genes were useful at an earlier stage in human history, when high-performance energy (quickly digestible carbohydrates) wasn't easy to come by. The fact of the matter is that glucose metabolism genes are common in nearly all living cells that have a nucleus (as opposed to bacteria, for example). We find examples of this mechanism in yeast, nematodes, fruit flies, mice, rats, and other mammals. So evolution has conserved it across many species for hundreds of millions of years.[*]

---

[*]The thrifty gene hypothesis does have its critics. If thrifty genes have been around for the 200,000 years or so that we *Homo sapiens* have existed, and agriculture began only around 12,000 years ago, pretty much everyone should carry the majority of the thrifty genes that have ever existed. Dr. John Speakman, a prominent challenger of the thrifty gene hypothesis, showed in a 2016 paper that none of the common obesity-related genes that had been identified conferred any properties or traits that could be considered to have provided an adaptive advantage. On the other hand, perhaps there are bona fide thrifty genes that will be identified with more advanced technology, so the case is not yet closed.

Because our genome since ancient times has had an average mutation rate of only 0.5 percent per million years, the nutritional requirements of humans must have been established by natural selection during the millions of years of our evolution. So let's go back in time and trace our origins from before *Homo sapiens* developed. In order to know what—and how—to eat, we need to understand the nutritional milieu in which the genetic makeup of our species was established.

TIMELINE OF HUMAN EVOLUTION[2]

55 million years ago (MYA)
The first primitive primates appear. They are small tree-dwelling creatures with monkey-like features.

8–6 MYA
The first gorillas appear. Later, the chimpanzee and human lineages diverge.

5.8 MYA
Orrorin tugenensis, the oldest human ancestor thought to have walked on two legs, appears.

5.5 MYA
Ardipithecus, an early protohuman that shares traits with chimps and gorillas and is forest dwelling, appears.

4 MYA

Australopithecines appear. They have brains no larger than a chimpanzee's, with a volume around 400–500 cubic centimeters (cc), but walk upright on two legs.

3.2 MYA

"Lucy," a famous specimen of *Australopithecus afarensis*, lives near what is now Hadar, Ethiopia.

2.7 MYA

Paranthropus, which lives in woods and grasslands and has massive jaws for chewing on roots and vegetation, makes an appearance. Becomes extinct 1.2 MYA.

2.5 MYA

Homo habilis emerges. Its face protrudes less than that of earlier hominids but still retains many apelike features. Has a brain volume of around 600 cc. Hominids regularly use stone tools, created by chipping pebbles; this starts the Oldowan tradition of toolmaking, which lasts a million years. Some hominids develop meat-rich diets as scavengers; it's thought that the extra energy fostered the evolution of larger brains.

2 MYA

Homo ergaster, with a brain volume of up to 850 cc, appears in Africa.

1.8–1.5 MYA

Homo erectus appears in Asia. It is the first true hunter-gatherer ancestor and also the first to have migrated out of Africa in large numbers. It attains a brain size of around 1,000 cc.

1.6 MYA

The possible first use of fire is suggested by discolored sediments in Koobi Fora, Kenya. More convincing evidence of charred wood and stone tools is found in Israel and dated to 780,000 years ago. Complex stone tools start to be produced and are the dominant technology until 100,000 years ago (YA).

600,000 YA

Homo heidelbergensis lives in Africa and Europe. It has a brain capacity similar to that of modern humans.

500,000 YA

The earliest evidence of purpose-built shelters—wooden huts—are found in sites near Chichibu, Japan.

400,000 YA

Early humans begin to hunt with spears.

325,000 YA

The oldest surviving human footprints are left by three people who clambered down the slopes of a volcano in Italy.

280,000 YA

The first complex stone blades and grinding stones appear.

230,000 YA

Neanderthals show up and are found across Europe, from Britain in the west to Iran in the east, until they become extinct with the entrance of modern humans 28,000 YA.

195,000 YA

Our own species, *Homo sapiens*, comes on the scene in Africa— and shortly thereafter begins to migrate across Asia and Europe. The oldest modern human remains are two skulls found in Ethiopia that date to this period. The average human brain volume is 1,350 cc.

170,000 YA

"Mitochondrial Eve," the direct ancestor of all living people today, may have been living in Africa.

150,000 YA

Humans are possibly capable of speech. 100,000-year-old shell jewelry suggests that they have developed complex speech and symbolism.

140,000 YA

The first evidence of long-distance trade appears.

110,000 YA

The earliest beads—made from ostrich egg shells—and jewelry are made.

50,000 YA

The "great leap forward": Human culture starts to change much more rapidly than before; people begin burying their dead ritually, creating clothes from animal hides, and developing complex hunting techniques such as pit traps. The colonization of Australia by modern humans occurs.

33,000 YA

The oldest known cave art is created. Later, Stone Age artisans create the spectacular murals at Lascaux and Chauvet in France. *Homo erectus* dies out in Asia, replaced by modern man.

18,000 YA

Homo floresiensis, "Hobbit" people, exist on the Indonesian island of Flores. They stand just over 1 meter tall and have brains similar in size to those of chimpanzees, yet have advanced stone tools.

12,000 YA

Modern people reach the Americas.

10,000 YA

Agriculture develops and spreads. The first villages arise. Possible domestication of dogs.

5,500 YA

The Stone Age ends and the Bronze Age begins. Humans begin to smelt and work copper and tin and use implements made of those metals in place of stone implements.

5,000 YA

The earliest known writing appears.

4,000–3,500 BCE

The Sumerians of Mesopotamia develop the world's first civilization.

EARLY HUMANS AS OMNIVORES: PLANT AND MEAT EATERS

In 2012, researcher Vincent Balter of the École Normale Supérieure de Lyon in France and his colleagues published a paper showing their analysis of various isotope patterns in tooth enamel in *Australopithecus africanus*, an ancestor of ours who lived between 3 million and 2 million years ago in a region of South Africa.[3] Female *A. africanus* members were about 3.9 feet tall and weighed about 60 pounds, whereas the males were up to 10 inches taller and 33 percent heavier. They had a diet similar to that of modern chimpanzees, consisting of fruit, plants, nuts, seeds, roots, insects, eggs, and some small-animal meat. From the *Australopithecus* group's descendants arose at least two separate branches. One was the *Paranthropus* group, which as *P. robustus* had very large teeth with thick enamel and large chewing muscles that allowed them to grind down tough, fibrous foods. They are not believed to be one of our direct ancestors but shared an ecological niche with early *Homo*, from which we are descended. The other was the *Homo* group, which produced *Homo habilis* ("handy man," possibly a direct ancestor) and later *Homo erectus* ("upright man," likely to have been a direct ancestor). *H. habilis* lived for about 1 million years, from 2.5 million to 1.4 million years ago. Though an omnivore like *A. africanus*, *H. habilis* started scavenging animal carcasses from under the noses of fearsome predators such as lions. Since they didn't possess fire, they couldn't eat the muscle meat, but they had a secret weapon: stone tools, which they used to smash open animal bones and skulls to extract the nutritious bone marrow and possibly the brains. Since *P. robustus* maintained his ancestors' brain size (400–500 cc) and *H. habilis* increased his brain size dramatically (to 600–900 cc), one can surmise that the need to obtain meat was the reason for that brain expansion.

Early African *H. erectus* fossils (dating from 1.89 million to roughly 143,000 to 70,000 years ago) are the oldest known early humans to have had modern humanlike body proportions with relatively elongated legs and shorter arms compared to the size of the torso. These attributes are adaptations to living on the ground, indicating the loss of earlier tree-climbing adaptations, with the ability to walk upright and possibly run long distances. They ranged in height from 4 feet, 9 inches to 6 feet, 1 inch and weighed 88 to 150 pounds. *H. erectus* was equipped with a large, thick skull, a large brain (900 cc on average), impressive brow ridges, and a strong, heavy body.

Scientists believe *H. erectus* was the first of many subsequent waves of humans to emigrate out of Africa into Eurasia. Since at that time they did not have the ability to make fire (they made use only of sporadically and serendipitously found fire), they originally settled no further than about 40 degrees north latitude. However, in that location, there are seasons during which plants don't grow and during which *H. erectus* had to rely solely on animals for food (especially raw bone marrow, organs, and fat, which are more digestible than muscle without using fire). Another indication that they were more like us than previous ancestors, fossil records show they cared for the old and weak individuals in their groups. By 500,000 years ago, *H. erectus* was intelligent and dexterous enough to use slim, smooth shells as tools and brainy enough to engrave an abstract pattern on at least one of them, probably using a shark's tooth as a tool. *H. erectus* produced large tools shaped by bifacial flaking, including hand axes. Hand axes are interpreted as tools associated with the butchering of large game. In recent years it has been suggested that *H. erectus* first used fire around 780,000 years ago; however, its use was rare and opportunistic until about 400,000 years ago, when they learned to make a fire and thus use it in daily cooking and other activities. It's then that we find them spreading throughout the even colder climates of northern Europe and Asia.

The next descendant of *H. erectus, Homo heidelbergensis,* was better adapted to the cold and roamed the globe from about 700,000 to 300,000 years ago. At Boxgrove, England, paleontologists found an abundance of tools made by them and bones from butchered large herbivores, including now-extinct species of rhinoceros and bears and smaller mammals such as voles (you read correctly—rhinoceros in England!). In the 1990s, in an old mine in Schöningen, Germany, Dr. Hartmut Thieme discovered eight wooden throwing spears. The weapons date from between 300,000 and 400,000 years ago. They also found about 16,000 bones, 90 percent of which were from horses, followed by red deer and European bison.

While the European *H. heidelbergensis* evolved into *Homo neanderthalensis* (aka Neanderthal) around 450,000 years ago, spreading throughout Europe and Asia, the African *H. heidelbergensis* group evolved into *Homo sapiens* ("wise man"—you and me) 300,000 to 200,000 years ago. Between 70,000 and 60,000 years ago, modern humans began their journey out of Africa, expanding into Eurasia and encountering their ancient cousins, including Neanderthals and Denisovans, both of whom we likely interbred with, but they mysteriously died out 20,000 to 30,000 years ago, leaving only us, *Homo sapiens*.

MODERN HUMANS

Not until 2003, when the mapping of the human genome was complete, did we really know that we're all related to one another (and we're even carrying a few percent of Neanderthal inherited genes). As mentioned before, since ancient times, our genome has had an average mutation rate of 0.5 percent per million years. We have not changed since the end of the Paleolithic era, and thus are living in the last 0.5 percent of human history. When humans began to move into Europe and Asia, they carried with them the genes that allowed us to survive in the African savanna, and only minor adaptions have taken place since then.

In comparison to the diet of preagricultural *Homo sapiens* living in the Upper Paleolithic period (40,000 to 10,000 years ago), also referred to as the Late Stone Age, the diet of contemporary humans has an overabundance of protein, simple sugars, sodium, and chloride and a paucity of fiber, calcium, and potassium. Is it really any wonder that we have an obesity epidemic and suffer from a wide spectrum of diseases rooted in diets our bodies weren't accustomed to eating? A large-scale study published in *The Journal of the American Medical Association* in 2019 showed that an increased consumption of high-glycemic, processed food is associated with a 14 percent increased risk of "all-cause mortality" (dying of anything).[4] Another study, also released in 2019, which I mentioned earlier, published in *The Lancet*, declared that globally, 1 in 5 deaths in 2017 were associated with poor nutrition.[5] This is twenty-first-century biological warfare that was unheard of among our ancestors.

All central Europeans were hunter-gatherers until around 7,500 years ago. They were the descendants of the first anatomically modern humans who survived the last Ice Age and arrived in Europe around 45,000 years ago. Genetic studies done by Professor Joachim Burger's group at the Institute of Anthropology at Johannes Gutenberg University Mainz in Germany indicate that agriculture and a sedentary lifestyle were brought to central Europe around 7,500 years ago by immigrant farmers.[6] From that time on, little trace of hunting-gathering can be seen in the archaeological record, and it is widely assumed that the hunter-gatherers died out or became part of the farming population.

Although we hear people today tout the "paleo diet" as if everyone should be eating that way, you might be surprised to learn that there is no such thing as a single "paleo diet." Our success as a species can be ascribed to our adaptability to whatever environment our ancestors settled in as they migrated away from their origins. In other words, the menu varied wildly. They ate what they could when they could based on what was available in their surroundings. A group of people in a coastal area would not have eaten the same as an inland group or as another group in a northern territory, where plant food was less available. But general patterns did exist from which we can create a framework. For the most part, a paleo diet is rich in high-quality protein and fat (though by saying "rich," I do not mean our ancestors ate "richly" every day), seasonal vegetables, legumes, fruits, and nuts. There are no highly refined or processed carbohydrates, little sugar, and no dairy products.

We know from the examination of human fossils that our Paleolithic ancestors were tall, enjoyed relatively good health, and were generally free of "modern" diseases such as cancer, heart disease, arthritis, and dental cavities (the so-called diseases of civilization).

THE LIFE SPAN OF HUNTER-GATHERERS

Besides the fact that it takes very favorable conditions to preserve bones so that they fossilize and are found by modern paleontologists—and thus bones are few and far between—it's also very difficult to gauge the age of any given individual from whom the bones came without having a large sample of bones with which to compare. Thus, certain bones could be those of a healthy 30-year-old or of a very healthy 60-year-old. We can't really compare them to bones from more modern times, when the environment and diet were substantially different. That's why looking at modern hunter-gatherer tribes can tell us a lot about the possible life span of our Paleolithic ancestors.

In 2007, Michael Gurven of UC Santa Barbara and Hillard Kaplan of the University of New Mexico published a paper titled "Longevity Among Hunter-Gatherers: A Cross-Cultural Examination."[7] In it, they attempted to summarize the most complete record available of high-quality demographic studies of contemporary hunter-gatherer populations. They concluded that there is a characteristic life span for our species, in which mortality—the risk of death—decreases sharply from infancy through childhood. This is followed by a period in which mortality rates remain essentially the same to about age 40, after which mortality rises steadily in Gompertz fashion.[*]

For humans, a line is crossed around the seventh decade. It's the line that separates the time when we are vigorous producers

---

[*]In 1825, an English actuary by the name of Benjamin Gompertz calculated the risk of death for people of different ages in order to determine how much to charge for life insurance. Using data from various parts of England, he found that the risk of death increased in a predictable way with age, which is not a surprise. Specifically, he concluded that the death rate doubled roughly every ten years between the ages of 20 and 60, which was the dominant age range for people buying insurance annuities at that time. The mathematical formula Gompertz used to predict the exponential rise in mortality after age 20 has become known colloquially as the Gompertz equation, and it has remained a fundamental part of mortality computations done by actuaries and demographers ever since the early nineteenth century.

and when senescence begins to set in, foreboding death. Scientists hypothesize that human bodies were designed to function well for about seven decades in the environment in which our species evolved. Although mortality rates differ among populations and among periods, especially in the risk of violent death, those differences are small in a comparative cross-species perspective. Gurven and Kaplan's calculations showed that individuals who survived until age 40 could expect to live an additional twenty-three to twenty-six years (to age 63–66), whereas if they made it to age 65, they could expect to live another five to ten years (to age 70–75), and so on. They found that premodern populations had an average modal adult life span of about 72 years, with a range of 68–78 years. "Modal age" refers to a peak in distribution of death, which nevertheless means that there's a variation in the ages to which a small number of individuals may live. Thus, before age 80, *most* hunter-gatherers would have died, but a very small percentage could have lived into their 90s or to 100 or beyond. This is not so far off the mortality rates for people in poor parts of the world today. And this fact goes against the conventional wisdom that says our ancestors didn't live long and that people in poor parts of the world today are doomed to an early death.

THE PALEO/HUNTER-GATHERER DIET

To get their daily calories, our ancestors would have focused on killing large game animals, such as elk, mastodons, mammoths, and now-extinct camels and horses. There are several reasons why they would have preferred eating fat over protein. First, fat has

9 calories per gram versus 4 calories per gram of protein. Sources of fat were plentiful on large animals, including bone marrow, organs, brain, and the fat surrounding muscle and organs. There's plenty of evidence from broken bones left in our ancestors' garbage pits that they ate marrow as often as they could. Second, uncooked meat is hard to chew and digest. Even after they learned how to use and later sustain fire as a means of cooking meat about 400,000 years ago, making it softer and more easily digestible, they ran into the problem that our bodies have a limit to how much protein they can process at a given time (remember this fact because it plays into the reason why we should limit our protein intake).

IDENTIFYING VARIOUS SOURCES OF PROTEIN

A new technology called liquid chromatography–isotope ratio mass spectrometry (LC-IRMS) began to be used about a decade ago, whereby through the measurement of carbon and nitrogen isotope ratios scientists can tell whether the proteins in collagen taken from human or animal bones were derived from a diet of primarily animals or plants. Herbivores' collagen displays different isotopic profiles from carnivores'. Scientists can even tell how high up the food chain the animal or human is, based on the concentration levels of these isotopes. Since the carbon ingested by marine animals (fish and shellfish) differs from the carbon ingested by terrestrial animals, this technology can also distinguish between proteins derived from consuming marine animals and those derived from consuming terrestrial animals.

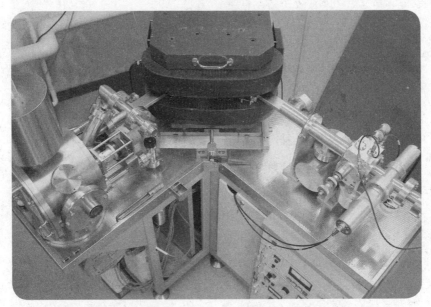

The machine that performs liquid chromatography-isotope ratio mass spectrometry.

Michael Richards, a paleobiologist formerly at the Max Planck Institute for Evolutionary Anthropology in Leipzig, Germany, has looked at thousands of bone samples in order to tell what various animals (including primates from our own lineage) were eating. In 2009, he published a paper with a Canadian anthropologist, Erik Trinkaus, reporting on the direct isotopic evidence for Neanderthal and early modern humans' diets in Europe.[8] They found that Neanderthals from about 120,000 to 37,000 years ago were top-level carnivores, obtaining all or most of their dietary protein from large herbivores, and there was no evidence of their eating marine foods. This finding is in agreement with analysis of Neanderthal tools and middens (garbage dumps where waste, including animal bones, human excrement, and so forth was left), as well as the local flora and fauna (all of the plants and animal fossils in a particular fossil layer). Unlike the Neanderthals, however, the early humans that Richards and Trinkaus studied ate not only terrestrial animals but a significant amount of marine animals.

Stanley Boyd Eaton is a Harvard-trained doctor and now retired diagnostic radiologist who worked most of his life in Atlanta, Georgia, where he specialized in musculoskeletal disorders (his patients often included members of the Atlanta Braves, the Atlanta Hawks, and the Atlanta Falcons). Dr. Eaton was one of the first doctors to write about Paleolithic nutrition. He published a number of papers with Melvin Konner, a PhD and colleague from Harvard who is a professor of anthropology and of neuroscience and behavioral biology at Emory University. One of the duos' seminal papers was "Paleolithic Nutrition—A Consideration of Its Nature and Current Implications," published in 1985 in the *The New England Journal of Medicine*.[9] It has been heavily cited in other papers since then.

According to Eaton and Konner, when the Cro-Magnons and other truly modern human beings appeared, concentration on big-game hunting increased; techniques and equipment were fully developed while the human population was still small in relation to the biomass of available game animals. In some areas during that time, animals probably provided over 50 percent of their diet. But because of overhunting, climate changes, and population growth, the period shortly before the inception of agriculture and animal husbandry was marked by a shift away from big-game hunting and toward a broader spectrum of subsistence activities. Remains of fish, shellfish, and small game are all more common at sites dating from that period, as well as tools that are useful for processing plant foods, such as grindstones, mortars, and pestles. In at least two Middle Eastern sites, trace element analysis for strontium levels in bone has revealed a definite increase in the amount of vegetable material in the diet together with decreased meat consumption. Modern hunter-gatherers most closely resemble the human beings of this relatively recent period.

Agriculture dramatically changed human nutritional patterns: over the course of a few millennia, the proportion of meat declined drastically, while vegetable foods came to make up as much as 90 percent of the diet. This shift resulted in significant consequences to the body's structure. Early European *Homo sapiens*, who ate an abundance of animal protein 30,000 years ago, were an average of 6 inches taller than their descendants who lived after the development of farming. The same pattern was repeated later in the New World. The Paleoindians were big-game hunters 10,000 years ago, but their descendants, who lived just before European contact, practiced intensive food production, ate little meat, were considerably shorter, and had skeletal manifestations that reflected suboptimal nutrition. The combination of the direct effects of protein calorie deficiency and the interaction between malnutrition and infection also had its impact. Since the Industrial Revolution, the protein content of Western diets has become more nearly adequate, and there's physical proof in an increase in average height. We are now nearly as tall as were the first biologically modern preagricultural human beings. But our diets still differ profoundly from theirs, and these differences lie at the heart of what has been termed "affluent malnutrition," which is causing the diseases of civilization.

AFFLUENT MALNUTRITION AND GENETIC MISMATCH

To say our diets are out of sync with our genetic evolutionary heritage is an understatement. The advent of agriculture led to dire outcomes in the health and welfare of many populations around the world. As I've been describing, our ancestors ate a good deal of high-fat meat, organ meats, and brains (also high in fat), freshwater fish and shellfish (rich in fatty acids), and fat from nuts and seeds, coconuts, and avocados. They preferred very fatty animals (mammoths, elephants, and hippopotami) to leaner game (deer and smaller game animals), which they fed to their dogs except when their supply of the fatter animals ran out.

With the advent of agriculture in southern Europe, as I just noted, the average height of the population decreased by 6 inches. The average longevity also took a dip, declining by ten years. Similar effects were observed in Native North Americans when agriculture was adopted a thousand years before Columbus discovered they were there. Holdouts against the agricultural trend, such as the nomadic cultures (e.g., Osage, Kiowa, Blackfeet, Shoshone, Assiniboine, and Lakota) that lived almost solely on the buffalo, were 6 to 12 inches taller than the European settlers, whose sustenance depended on wheat and corn. Interestingly, the Masai in East Africa also lived as nomadic herders on a diet of meat and milk, and they, too, were known for their unusual height and physical prowess. Also, even in the early 1900s, the inhabitants of remote northeastern Canada had almost no heart disease, cancer, or Alzheimer's disease. However, those living near "civilization" who ingested flour and sugar had all of these diseases.

Although the Agricultural Revolution started more than 10,000 years ago, refined carbohydrates (sugar and white flour) didn't make it into most people's diets until the Middle Ages. Throughout the 1800s, Western doctors were sent by their governments to work with "native populations," and they documented how quickly those people changed from healthy, lean hunter-gatherers to obese individuals subject to the same diseases of civilization—cancer, heart disease, hypertension, type 2 diabetes, obesity, dental cavities, autoimmune diseases, osteoporosis, Alzheimer's disease, and so on—as Westerners, as they were provided with more and more flour and sugar. In the early 1800s, the average American consumed only about 15 pounds of sugar a year (there may not have been vending machines filled with sugary treats and cereals, but sugar has been around since sugarcane was first cultivated thousands of years ago, followed by other sources of sugar). By the end of the twentieth century, consumption had grown nearly tenfold and Americans were consuming, on average, at least 120 pounds of sugar a year per person![10] A well-developed refrigeration and transportation infrastructure meant, too, that dairy products became a daily staple in everyone's lives. As we've previously learned, these lifestyle changes resulted in higher blood glucose and branched-chain amino acid (BCAA) levels, keeping people's switch turned up for mTOR and down for autophagy, twenty-four hours a day, seven days a week.

JAMES W. CLEMENT

THE ABSENCE OF DAIRY PRODUCTS, GRAINS, PROCESSED SUGARS, VEGETABLE OILS, AND ALCOHOL IN EARLY DIETS

According to Colorado State University Professor Emeritus Loren Cordain, who is often credited as being a founder of the modern "paleo movement," implements for grinding cereal grains first appeared in the Upper Paleolithic, from about 40,000 to 12,000 years ago, but evidence of the regular and sustained exploitation of cereal grains by any worldwide hunter-gatherer group arose with the emergence of the Natufian culture in the Levant in the eastern Mediterranean region about 13,000 years ago.[11] Animals were not domesticated before 11,000 to 10,000 years ago, but there isn't reliable evidence of milk being collected for consumption before 6,000 years ago. Honey appears to have been a small part of any hunter-gatherer's diet, and crystalline sucrose production from sugarcane didn't appear until about 2,500 years ago, in India. Olive oil was one of the first man-made oils, dating back to about 6,000 years ago. Other oils for consumption were virtually unheard of until the Industrial Revolution of the late 1800s made processing on a mass scale feasible. The first fermentation of wine likely occurred about 7,500 years ago, and the brewing of cereal grains into beer first took place about 4,000 years ago. Distilling of alcoholic beverages didn't occur until about 1,200 years ago. As you can see, these food sources, which collectively make up nearly three-quarters of current American calorie intake, were only recently introduced into our diets, and it's unlikely that most of us have genetically adapted to these foods.

Bear in mind that the transition from a hunter-gatherer dietary lifestyle has varied geographically and wasn't the norm in northern Europe, England, or Scotland until about 2,000 to 1,500 years ago. Furthermore, refined carbohydrates, grain-fed animals, and simple sugars, all now in abundance in Western diets, have been widely available for only 100 to 150 years. No one's going to argue that that's enough time for people to have adapted to these foods.

The transition from a hunter-gatherer-based to a cereal-based diet resulted in numerous detrimental health effects: increased infant mortality, lower height, less bone density, more dental decay, increased anemia, and reduced life span.

LOW-GLYCEMIC, HIGH-FIBER FOODS IN EARLY DIETS

There's evidence that *Homo* has been eating seeds, grasses, berries, and other low-glycemic, high-fiber vegetables, fruits, and "resistant starches" (such as true yams and taro root) for a very long time. Researchers from the Smithsonian Institution and the Center for Advanced Study of Hominid Paleobiology at George Washington University in Washington, DC, analyzed dental tartar from the mouths of circa 44,000-year-old Neanderthal skull fossils and found that their owners had apparently eaten a variety of plant foods, including date palms, legumes, and grass seeds, some of which involved cooking.

But because such foods don't supply much in the way of calories, the bulk of their daily calorie intake would still have been animal meat (protein) and fat throughout much of every year. Don't forget, those guys were bigger and more active than average present-day humans, and they would have had caloric needs similar to ours: 1,800 calories per day for women and up to 2,800 calories per day for men. One and a half cups of spinach (about 13 ounces) provides only 100 calories, although this low-glycemic green vegetable provides about 12 grams of fiber.

A lot of modern processed foods are fortified, which the manufacturers tell us is a good thing (after all, the word "fortified" implies an increase in nutritive value—a food made stronger). But here's something you probably haven't heard before: the overconsumption of food products that are fortified with niacin (vitamin B_3) may also increase the risk of certain conditions. In the early 2000s, the US daily per capita consumption of niacin exceeded 33 milligrams, twice the RDA set by the US Food and Nutrition Board. Large doses of niacin have long been known to impair glucose tolerance, induce insulin resistance, and enhance insulin release.[12] Niacin is also a potent stimulator of appetite, whereas niacin deficiency may lead to appetite loss, meaning that it ties directly into one's ability to lose weight. According to researchers in China and Japan, niacin derived from grain products exceeded the amount derived from meat in the United States in the early 1970s, due primarily to an update of niacin fortification standards that required manufacturers to put more niacin into their products.[13]

(As an aside: Niacin is turned into NAD+ and used by the mitochondria to make ATP, or cellular energy. However, it converts to NAD+ very poorly. With the help of a physician and various other collaborators, I've been conducting a series of clinical trials to determine how to increase NAD+ through other means, such as direct infusions of NAD+ or oral consumption of the precursor nicotinamide riboside. This keeps various longevity genes turned on while reducing the buildup of nicotinamide that comes with excess niacin consumption, especially as we age.)

THE PERILS OF OUR MODERN DIET

Jared Diamond, an acclaimed geographer, Pulitzer Prize–winning author, and one of the world's leading historians, has written extensively on the impact of agriculture on human health. He was one of the first to document changes in height and longevity with the advent of agriculture, calling it "the worst mistake in the history of the human race."[14] Not only has he written about how hunter-gatherers enjoyed a highly variable diet, in contrast to early farmers, but he has pointed out that the trade facilitated by the Agricultural Revolution may have contributed to the spread of germs and infectious diseases. He boldly states that the adoption of agriculture, "supposedly our most decisive step toward a better life, was in many ways a catastrophe from which we have never recovered."[15] The historian Yuval Noah Harari doubled down on this idea in his best-selling *Sapiens: A Brief History of Humankind*: "The Agricultural Revolution certainly enlarged the sum total of food at the disposal of humankind, but the extra food did not translate into a better diet or more leisure. . . . The Agricultural Revolution was history's biggest fraud."[16]

Our move away from a hunter-gatherer lifestyle and toward agriculture-based subsistence had its merits. It's partially responsible for the swift rise in population growth and the establishment of more stable communities. But although we increased in number, our diets did not necessarily become healthier. Farming fostered an abundance of food, and as a result, we could easily consume more calories than we needed. Moreover, farming also led to a less diverse diet, especially once we began to generate processed cereal- and grain-based food products filled with artificial and refined ingredients. Some have argued that agriculture changed the course of our history more than any other human-driven event. And with the absence of diet diversity came a dearth of nutrients, too. The combination of nutrient deficiency and a bounty of calorie-dense refined foods always available meant we grew heavier, wider, and sicker. According to researchers at Tufts University, "prescribing" whole foods—fruits and vegetables—would save $100 billion in medical costs each year in the United States alone.[17]

Now let's turn to the more granular part of the conversation and understand what's going on biologically as we consume more agriculture-based, processed foods to the detriment of our health.

SPACE AGE GENES IN A STONE AGE WORLD

If you could be transported to Paleolithic times, you would be hard-pressed to run into a lot of obese people. The disconnect or mismatch between our ancient physiology and the Western diet and lifestyle has been deemed the result of living in the Space Age with Stone Age genes. It's the Flintstones meet the Jetsons. If you were to compare the bodies of two people who have the same height and bone structure, but one weighs a lean 120 pounds and another is 250 pounds, they would look totally different from the outside. A scan would show the same skeletal frame within both of them, yet one is saddled with lots of extra fat.

The "thrifty gene" hypothesis suggests that the difference between those two people reflects an obvious mismatch between our Stone Age genes and Space Age environment. We all know someone who can eat a large volume of food at meals, yet remain extraordinarily lean (and may not even be a regular exerciser). But that person probably would not have survived long in the Stone Age. Such people, whom we view as fortunate today, are the opposite of the thrifty phenotype. A person who easily gains weight no matter what he or she eats retains more of the foods' calories in the form of fat. He or she will survive much longer under conditions of starvation. Being able to effectively store excess consumed energy helped us survive in our evolution. That worked well for the millions of years during which our ancestors faced scarce resources, but it has become a problem for bodies designed for scarcity in modern times of relative caloric abundance, and overconsumption can result in ending up overweight or obese.

An important biological concept to grasp is that not everyone burns calories equally and not all calories are created equal. Calories in food are measured using what is called a bomb calorimeter, which determines the heat of combustion through the ignition of a sample in pure oxygen at high pressure in a sealed vessel and the measurement of the resulting rise in temperature. Technically, a calorie is the energy needed to raise the temperature of 1 gram of water 1°C (one dietary calorie contains 4,184 joules of energy). But the human body is not like a bomb calorimeter. It does not burn calories the same way a bomb calorimeter does. A calorie is a calorie only if you are trying to boil water. Recall that I said protein provides about 4 calories per gram, while fat provides 9 calories per gram (clearly, fats are more energy dense). But biologically speaking, proteins, carbohydrates (which also provide 4 calories per gram), and fats are vastly different because each is metabolized differently and under some circumstances your body favors storing one and burning the other and vice versa.

The way your body responds to consuming 100 calories of carbohydrates in the form of refined sugar (about 6 teaspoons of granulated pure cane sugar) will not be the same as when you consume 100 calories of fat in the form of olive oil (about 1 tablespoon). You can even feel the difference in your hunger cues and level of satiety. You can easily attune yourself to this fact by performing a little experiment. One day, have a carb-centric breakfast, such as a Belgian waffle with syrup or a bowl of cereal (any kind) with nonfat milk, and see how long you can go without feeling hungry and eating again. The next day, eat a fat-heavy breakfast with protein, such as a vegetable frittata. Try to ensure that both meals contain the same number of calories. The waffle or cereal breakfast will leave most people ready to eat again within a couple of hours or less. The egg plate will likely keep you satisfied for several hours. Your body didn't metabolize the breakfasts in the same way, even though they contain the same amount of energy. And you experienced each meal differently. So what's going on to explain this discrepancy? A lot.

Eating and metabolizing nutrients is a complex phenomenon. You're setting in motion a multitude of hormonal pathways that affect how your food is digested, how your cells react, how your brain interprets hunger and satiety signals, and eventually, how you feel. If we all used calories the same way, we would never see a vast spectrum of differences among us in the ability to maintain a certain weight with the same dietary intake and physical output. No two metabolisms are exactly the same.

THE PROBLEM WITH SUGAR

In 2011, Gary Taubes, the author I mentioned earlier who wrote *Good Calories, Bad Calories* and *Why We Get Fat*, wrote a popular essay for the *New York Times* titled "Is Sugar Toxic?"[18] In it, he chronicled not just the history of sugar in our lives and food products, but the evolving science behind understanding how sugar affects our bodies. This was followed by *The Case Against Sugar* in late 2016, in which he accused sugar of being the main cause of chronic diseases.[19] Robert Lustig, a specialist in pediatric hormone disorders and a leading expert in childhood obesity at the University of California, San Francisco, School of Medicine has also written extensively on this topic (Taubes cites Lustig's work as well). According to Lustig, who wrote *Fat Chance: Beating the Odds Against Sugar, Processed Food, Obesity, and Disease*, the body metabolizes various types of sugars differently.[20] Pure glucose, the simplest form of sugar, is not the same as white granulated table sugar, which is a combination of glucose and fructose. (Fructose, which I'll get to shortly, is a type of naturally occurring sugar found exclusively in fruit and honey; it is the sweetest of all naturally occurring carbohydrates.) Gram for gram, the two types of sugar provide the same number of calories. But they are processed differently by the body. Here's what happens.

As you've already learned, glucose raises blood sugar and can be metabolized by all of your body's cells. Fructose, on the other hand, is received a little differently by the body. When you consume it, it's handled exclusively by your liver and has no immediate effect on your insulin level. Drinking liquid fructose, such as that found in juice and soda, is not the same as consuming an equivalent amount in the form of whole fruit or honey. Fructose has the lowest glycemic index of all the natural sugars. Although it may not trigger an immediate spike in blood sugar, fructose can have more long-term effects if it's overly consumed, especially from unnatural sources—the most notorious of which is high-fructose corn syrup. The science has long been established: consuming fructose is associated with impaired glucose tolerance, insulin resistance, high blood fat levels, and hypertension (high blood pressure). Fructose in excess is uniquely offensive to our metabolism in the sense that it does not trigger the production of insulin and leptin, two hormones that are key to regulating our metabolism and feelings of fullness or hunger. Which helps explain why a diet high in fructose can lead to obesity and its metabolic consequences.

Our Paleolithic ancestors ate fruit, but certainly not every day or even every month of the year, and the fruit they came across when the season was right was not nearly as sweet as the kind we cultivate and buy today. Our bodies are behind the times; we haven't yet evolved to be able to handle the large volume of fructose we down today, most of which is coming from manufactured sources far from nature. Natural fruit has relatively little sugar when compared to, say, a can of fructose-sweetened soda, which has a massive amount. Take, for example, a medium-size apple versus a 12-ounce can of fructose-sweetened soda. The apple has about 44 calories of sugar but it's held in a fiber-rich environment. There's soluble pectin fiber in the apple's flesh and insoluble fiber in the skin. The soda, on the other hand, contains approximately 80 calories of sugar—nearly twice the amount and no fiber whatsoever. Now, what happens when you create apple juice from a batch of apples, concentrating the liquid down to a 12-ounce beverage? You get a drink that is just about the same in terms of fructose and calories as the soda. And when that fructose reaches the liver, most of it is converted to fat and stored in our fat cells. For decades, biochemists have called fructose the most fattening carbohydrate! Think about what happens when our bodies have to do this conversion at every meal. At some point, our muscle tissue becomes resistant to insulin as well.

As mentioned, the majority of the fructose we consume is not in its natural form. The average American downs 163 grams of refined sugar (more than 650 calories' worth) per day, and of this, roughly 76 grams (more than 30 calories' worth) are from the highly processed form of fructose, derived from high-fructose corn syrup.[21] High-fructose corn syrup is the sugar that dominates in modern processed foods. Although you'll typically find statistics that indicate high-fructose corn syrup is comprised of about 55 percent fructose, 42 percent glucose, and 3 percent other carbohydrates, these percentages can vary tremendously by product. Studies have shown that high-fructose corn syrup can contain much more free fructose than labeled. Dr. Michael Goran, the director of the Childhood Obesity Research Center and professor of preventive medicine at the University of Southern California, identified levels of free fructose as high as 65 percent in soda purchased in the Los Angeles area.[22] Translation: You don't know what you're eating when you devour processed foods loaded with high-fructose corn syrup. And I'm not talking solely about junk foods, candy, and soda. This sugar can even lurk in unsuspecting places like condiments, salad dressings, energy bars, yogurts, and breads. It's everywhere today.

High-fructose corn syrup is a relatively recent addition to our diets. It was introduced in 1978 as a cheap replacement for table sugar in beverages and food products. You probably have already heard that it's a big culprit in our obesity epidemic, but high-fructose corn syrup is not the only character in the story. Though it's true we can partly accuse our consumption of high-fructose corn syrup of giving us big waistlines and diagnoses of related conditions such as metabolic syndrome, we can also point to *all other sugars* as well since they are *all carbohydrates*. These were not available with the touch of a button or swipe of a finger when our genes were evolving. I should also point out that other man-made chemicals often accompany high-fructose corn syrup in processed foods, and some of those chemicals can also be fat-inducing.[23]

I am describing all of this "sugar biology" because it helps explain how we can suffer so mightily today from diseases of civilization *in the absence of any underlying genetic propensity*. Sure, some people are genetically prone to develop diabetes, heart disease, or cancer. But I'd argue that all of us are vulnerable to these diseases if we push the *H. sapiens* metabolism and physiology over the proverbial cliff. And for all of you out there who inherited "bad genes" for a certain demise, let me also say that you can avert that fate through lifestyle. It cuts both ways. We all know people who live with a higher risk of developing an ailment that "runs in the family," or perhaps they are even diagnosed with gene variants related to a disease. But they never go on to develop the malady. A whole area of study today looks into the interaction between lifestyle factors and genetic expression in health span. It's called epigenetics, and scientists like Steve Horvath at UCLA are developing ways to measure the body's "epigenetic clock," which would indicate the body's biological age.

Lung cancer would probably be a much rarer disease if there were no tobacco industry. Similarly, obesity would likely be uncommon if there were no processed food industry that sold a lot of refined carbs. Other conditions such as diabetes, heart disease, dementia, and many cancers would probably be rare as well. I think it's time to use our ancestors as models and adopt a paleo-like healthy eating pattern—but with a twist.

EAT ACCORDING TO YOUR ANCESTRAL GENOME

Given the evolutionary history I described in this chapter, you can see how dysfunctional we are in our eating habits today. And we're not undergoing the vagaries of nomadic life, having to forage and hunt for food and suffer through famines. If we want to eat according to how our genome expects us to eat but at the same time leverage the power of autophagy, we can't be eating high levels of carbohydrates (refined flours and sugars especially) and animal protein daily. Even though our ancestors' diets were rooted in protein and fat, they were not consuming these macronutrients at every meal and snack as we do today! Far from it. We have to no longer eat like industrialists.

Though paleo diets are excellent at cutting out some of the worst-offending refined carbohydrates (especially refined flours and sugars), they still allow copious amounts of fruit year-round, honey, and of course lots of animal protein. These diets often encourage a much higher consumption of protein than would be desirable in order to keep mTOR turned down and autophagy turned up. This combination of too much carbs and protein, which several study authors call "nutrient overload," leads the followers of these diets to the diseases of civilization as surely as does a typical Western diet. In chapter 9, I'll be recommending foods that can fit into a paleo meal plan while still keeping mTOR in check.

CHAPTER 7

WALNUTS AND CORN-FED COWS

A s I've pointed out in previous chapters, consuming too many refined carbohydrates and too much animal protein will keep mTOR turned on all the time, resulting in your metabolic switch being stuck in the "growth" mode and keeping your intracellular housecleaning mechanism—autophagy—perpetually turned off. As I've also discussed, a high-fat diet can be the solution to maintaining your needed calorie intake while trimming your consumption of mTOR-activating refined carbohydrates and animal proteins (e.g., cheeseburgers, pizzas, Bolognese pasta, and steak and potatoes).

But thinking about a high-fat diet might conjure up vivid images of unhealthiness, greasy foodstuffs, and gluttony. As we've seen, burning fat is what powered our ancestors from the most remote caveman to your great-great-grandparents. Healthy levels of body fat provided a megastorehouse of energy for them to rely on in tough times, such as during the Irish potato famine or the American dust bowl during the Great Depression. It's a basic component of our bodies, in our muscle tissue, brain, and cell membranes. But as we're all painfully aware, an increasing number of us carry too much fat around. Back in the 1980s and '90s, when "fat free" became a popular marketing claim on foods, little did we know that the fat-free way of life (whereby fats were replaced mostly with refined flours and sugars) would have the opposite of its intended effect and lead us down a dangerous path to diabetes and obesity, especially when excess fat becomes lodged deep in our tissues and around vital organs. Visceral adipose tissue (aka VAT) is commonly called belly fat. It's found inside your abdominal cavity and wraps around your internal organs.

Belly fat is the worst because it has the most metabolic consequences, one of which happens when fat cells become *senescent*: they cease to divide but refuse to die off. Senescent cells give off pro-inflammatory signals that tell the immune system to mobilize, and when there are lots of senescent fat cells, this turns into chronic systemic inflammation. Because belly fat builds up around our organs, the pro-inflammatory signals from senescent fat cells wreak havoc with the proper functioning of those organs as well as causing stem cells to become dormant. And when stem cells, which are precursor baby-like cells that can differentiate into any type of cell, go dormant, trouble looms. The body can't use them to regenerate or repair diseased tissue and organs. Constant inflammation also overexcites your immune system, sometimes leading to autoimmune problems such as rheumatoid arthritis, multiple sclerosis, inflammatory bowel disease, and lupus.

Welcome to the fat chapter. I'm going to talk about good fats and bad fats, because if you're like most people, you've likely been getting the wrong facts or are completely confused by the contradictory claims by proponents of various diets or food marketers as to what makes you fat and what's healthy. When you have the right balance of dietary fat, you put yourself into a position to turn on autophagy more effectively.

FAT FUNDAMENTALS

Let's start with the basics. When we talk about fat as being uniquely critical for the body, most of the time we're referring to fatty acids, important chemical compounds found in plants, animals, and microorganisms. In humans, fatty acids help control blood pressure and inflammation and keep blood from clotting. They are the molecules that help with cellular development and the formation of healthy cell membranes, and they have been shown to block tumor formation in animals, as well as hinder the growth of human breast cancer cells.

I'll keep the chemistry lecture brief, but I do want you to gain a basic understanding about fat. (Unless you're a doctor, you probably learned some of this a long time ago and took one test on it.) A fatty acid typically consists of carbon atoms attached to each other in a straight chain with hydrogen atoms bound to the carbon atoms along the length of the chain, as well as at one end. At the other end is a carboxyl group (–COOH), and it's this carboxyl group that makes it an acid (carboxylic acid). The structure of these bonds determines whether the fatty acid is saturated or unsaturated. When the bonds linking the carbon atoms are all single, the fatty acid is said to be saturated; if any of the bonds is double or triple, the fatty acid is called unsaturated. A few fatty acids have branched chains (not to be confused with branched-chain amino acids [BCAAs], which are abundant in animal protein); others, such as prostaglandins (hormonelike fatty compounds that participate in smooth muscle contraction and relaxation), contain ring structures. Complicating this picture further, I must also add that fatty acids are found in combination with the alcohol glycerol in the form of triglyceride. The most widely distributed fatty acid is oleic oil, which is abundant in some vegetable oils (e.g., olive, palm, peanut, and sunflower seed) and makes up about 46 percent of body fat. In addition, there's the essential versus nonessential fatty acids. As their name implies, fatty acids that we need for survival but cannot make ourselves are called essential fatty acids; we must obtain them from our diet. Omega-3 and omega-6 fatty acids are the two biggest categories of essential fatty acids (much more on these shortly).

When we talk about dietary fats, we often refer to the three types: saturated fats, unsaturated fats, and trans fats. Saturated fats are usually solid at room temperature and are naturally found in animal meats and whole dairy products such as milk, cheese, butter, and cream. Some saturated fats are also found in plant foods such as tropical oils (coconut or palm) and nuts. They are the only fatty acids that raise total blood cholesterol levels and low-density lipoprotein (LDL, or "bad" cholesterol). For this reason, they may increase your risk of developing cardiovascular disease and type 2 diabetes if you consume too much of them and have an underlying genetic predisposition to those ailments. Although we tend to think of saturated fats as being "bad," every cell in your body requires them for survival. Your cells' membranes, in fact, are comprised of 50 percent saturated fats, contributing to the structure and function of your lungs, heart, bones, liver, and immune system. Even your endocrine system relies on saturated fatty acids to communicate the need to manufacture certain hormones, including insulin. And they help you put down your fork, telling your brain when you are full.

Trans fats are basically man-made synthetic fats that act similar to saturated fats. They are produced when corn, soybean, or vegetable oil is made into a solid fat through a process called hydrogenation (hence the phrases "hydrogenated oil" and "partially hydrogenated oil" on ingredients lists). Although trans fats are increasingly being phased out of a lot of manufactured food products thanks to the Food and Drug Administration's new policies, they still hide in many processed foods such as snack foods (crackers and chips), commercially baked goods (muffins, cookies, and cakes), shortening, and many fried fast-food items. These are probably the most pernicious and have hardly any redeeming properties, and my hope is that they will be obliterated from the food supply within a few years.

Unsaturated fats are usually liquid at room temperature. We find these in most vegetable products, nuts, and oils and they are often categorized as being monounsaturated or polyunsaturated. (Monounsaturated fats have one pair of carbon molecules linked by a double bond; polyunsaturated fats have two or more double bonds between carbon atoms in the carbon chain backbone of the fat.) Studies show that eating foods rich in monounsaturated fatty acids (MUFAs) improves blood cholesterol levels.[1] Research also shows that MUFAs may positively impact insulin and blood sugar levels, two excellent outcomes for controlling weight and the risk of developing metabolic dysfunction.[2] MUFAs include olive and canola oil, as well as avocados and the oil derived from them.* Polyunsaturated fatty acids (PUFAs) are found mostly in plant-based foods and oils, as well as in oils from fatty fish such as salmon, herring, halibut, and marine algae. Evidence shows that eating foods rich in PUFAs also improves blood cholesterol levels and may help decrease the risk of developing type 2 diabetes.[3] Omega-3 fatty acids are one type of polyunsaturated fat that may be especially protective.

The two key omega-3s we often hear about are docosahexae-noic acid (DHA) and eicosapentaenoic acid (EPA). We need both of these, although DHA gets more attention than EPA in its health-supporting role. (We need at least 200 to 300 milligrams daily, but most Americans consume less than 25 percent.) DHA is a major structural component of the mammalian brain and is the most abundant omega-3 fatty acid in the brain, which is why it's often touted for its brain-enhancing powers and apparent ability to reduce risk for cognitive decline and dementia. As the omega-3 fatty acid DHA is a prominent component of neuronal mem-branes, and as the human body is inefficient in synthesizing DHA, we are reliant on dietary DHA from fatty fish and DHA-enriched eggs.

Some of the mechanisms by which DHA affects the brain and

---

*Canola oil gets a bad reputation in popular health media. It can be overly processed and it does not wear as big of a health halo hat as olive oil. But because it has a higher smoke point, it can be the better option for high-heat cooking. Choose a quality organic brand.

cognition are starting to be elucidated in scientific research. For example, DHA dietary supplementation has been found to elevate levels of hippocampal brain-derived neurotrophic factor (BDNF, a brain growth hormone) and enhance cognitive function in rodents with brain trauma. Numerous studies, in fact, have shown a correlation between DHA levels and brain volume. In 2014, a large study assessed more than 1,100 postmenopausal women enrolled in the Women's Health Initiative Memory Study.[4] As with many of these studies, the researchers used MRI brain scans to measure brain volume at the beginning of the study and eight years later. Higher levels of DHA equated with a bigger brain, specifically the size of the hippocampus, which is the brain's memory center. An earlier 2012 study documented the same results upon examining more than 1,500 men and women who were part of the famous Framingham Heart Study.[5] (This has been among our most prized long-term studies in science, adding volumes of data to our understanding of certain risk factors for disease; it began in 1948 with the recruitment of 5,209 healthy men and women between the ages of 30 and 62 from the town of Framingham, Massachusetts. Researchers have followed them since, looking for clues to physiological conditions within the context of parameters such as age, gender, physical traits, and genetic patterns.[6])

So if you want to stave off the brain's natural shrinkage with age, consuming more DHA is one interventional strategy. It's thought that DHA enhances cognitive abilities by facilitating the brain's plasticity, which again is the brain's ability to rewire and reshape itself for the better. It fortifies connections and streamlines communication among brain cells. It might also act through its positive effects on metabolism, as it stimulates glucose utilization and mitochondrial function, thereby reducing oxidative stress. All of these effects help dial up autophagy when other conditions are in place, such as intermittent fasting, calorie restriction, and protein cycling.

Now, here's what's really important. One theory as to why DHA can be so brain friendly and support cognition is that when there's sufficient DHA in the diet, it becomes a vital ingredient in our cells' membranes, especially neurons in the brain. But when DHA is lacking, cells will incorporate other molecules, such as omega-6 fatty acids, into the membrane, even though they're vastly less flexible and hinder the transfer of electrical impulses entering the cell. Also, this substitution may affect structures called G-proteins that sit on the inside of the cell membrane and are a vital link in the transmission of signals among brain cells. These proteins help molecules on the outside of the membrane communicate with molecules on the inside.

The other omega-3 fatty acid component, EPA, is an important regulator of inflammation, and it appears to be particularly important for controlling cellular inflammation in the brain. In this realm, a lot of research on brain-related ailments such as depression, ADHD, and brain trauma have shown EPA to be superior to DHA. So you see, we do need both, and they often come together in foods and supplements.

Technically, cholesterol isn't always considered to be a fat, although it's just as important. Cholesterol is a waxy, soft, fat-like substance that every cell has the capacity to make. Contrary to what you might think, the two types of cholesterol you hear about, HDL (high-density lipoprotein) and LDL (low-density lipoprotein), are not two different kinds of cholesterol. HDL and

LDL are two different *vessels* for cholesterol and fats, and they each serve a unique biological role. We can't live without either LDL or HDL, but imbalances can arise. Having a low LDL level reduces the risk of developing heart disease and too much HDL can cause clogged or blocked arteries. In general, cholesterol forms cell membranes with other saturated fats. It also acts as a gatekeeper, helping to guard those membranes and supervise their permeability so various chemical reactions can take place both inside and outside the cell. The gallbladder's bile salts, for example, which are released to digest fat and facilitate the absorption of fat-soluble vitamins, are made of cholesterol. We often hear about the benefits of having low cholesterol. But you wouldn't want to be too low because that could compromise not only your ability to digest fat but also your body's electrolyte balance, which is managed partly by cholesterol.

Cholesterol also supports brain function and development. Your brain is only 2 percent of your body's total mass but it contains 25 percent of your total cholesterol. One-fifth of the brain by weight is cholesterol, and now we know why this may be so: the availability of cholesterol in the brain may determine whether or not we can grow new synapses (neural connections). Cholesterol is what brings brain cell membranes together so that signals can easily jump across the linking synapse. Cholesterol in the brain also serves as a powerful antioxidant. It protects the brain against the damaging effects of free radicals. Without cholesterol in the body, you wouldn't be able to produce steroid hormones such as estrogen and the androgens, as well as vitamin D, a critically important fat-soluble antioxidant. Cholesterol is a precursor molecule—a starter ingredient—in these hormones.

In addition to helping provide structure and function to various parts of the body, one of the chief reasons to consume dietary fat is to help absorb and use essential fat-soluble vitamins such as A, D, E, and K. "Fat-soluble" means these vitamins do not dissolve in water—they need fat around to be absorbed. If you lack vitamin K, you'd lack the ability to form blood clots and could suffer from spontaneous bleeding (this is the vitamin that newborns are given immediately after birth to prevent a potentially fatal, but rare, bleeding disorder). A deficiency of vitamin A would leave you vulnerable to blindness and infections. And a lack of vitamin D is known to be associated with increased susceptibility to several chronic diseases, including depression, neurodegenerative diseases, and a number of autoimmune diseases, such as type 1 diabetes; it may also increase the risk of developing heart diseases, especially hypertension and heart enlargement. It doesn't help that the American diet is already vitamin poor due to an overabundance of refined, unnatural foods; when we avoid eating fat, we put ourselves at even more risk of suffering from vitamin deficiencies.

THE FAT PARADOX

There are several legendary paradoxes whereby communities of people consume a lot of fat but never suffer the stereotypical consequences. In the Inuit's Nunavik villages in northern Quebec, for example, adults over 40 get almost half of their calories from native foods, which come largely from wild animals that range freely and eat what nature (rather than concentrated animal feeding operations, or CAFOs) intended.[7] More than 50 percent of their calorie intake is from fat, and they don't die of heart attacks at nearly the same rates as other Canadians or Americans. Their cardiac death rate is about half of ours. Their diets no doubt help them support autophagy to prevent disease.[8]

It's important to note that there's a big difference between fat from a wild animal and fat from a domesticated one.[9] Less of a wild animal's fat is saturated, and more of it is in the monounsaturated form (like that in olive oil). Wild game contains over five times more polyunsaturated fat per gram than is found in domestic livestock. Further, the fat of wild animals contains an appreciable amount (approximately 4 percent) of the omega-3 fatty acid EPA. As I covered earlier, this fatty acid is currently under clinical investigation because of its apparent anti-atherosclerotic, anti-inflammatory, and pro-cognition properties. Domestic (USDA-certified) beef, on the other hand, contains almost undetectable amounts of this important nutrient. Mass-produced USDA-certified beef comes from cattle fed a concentrated diet of grain, soy, corn, and other supplements. They are often also given growth hormones and antibiotics. This diet changes the natural composition of the meat they produce, resulting in beef that contains more calories gram for gram than does grass-fed beef, as well as a less favorable balance of healthy fats.

What's more, cold-water fish and sea mammals, also part of the Inuit diet, are particularly rich in polyunsaturated omega-3 fatty acids. As noted, these fats appear to benefit the heart and vascular system. But the polyunsaturated fats that make up the vast majority of most Americans' diets are the largely pro-inflammatory omega-6 fatty acids supplied in high quantities by vegetable oils, and most legumes, nuts, and seeds. By contrast, whale blubber consists of 70 percent monounsaturated fat and close to 30 percent omega-3s.

Omega-3s evidently help raise HDL cholesterol and lower triglycerides, and they are known for their anticlotting effects. (Ethnographers have remarked on Eskimos' propensity to nosebleeds.) These fatty acids are also believed to protect the heart from life-threatening arrhythmias that can lead to sudden cardiac death. And, like a "natural aspirin," omega-3 polyunsaturated fats help put the brakes on runaway inflammatory processes, which play a part in atherosclerosis, diabetes, obesity, arthritis, dementia, and other so-called diseases of civilization.[10]

As early as 1908, the Danish doctors (and married couple) August Krogh and Marie Krogh studied the Greenlandic Eskimo diet.[11] They demonstrated that Greenlanders were the population with the highest consumption of meat known at the time. Later, another pair of Danish doctors, Hans Olaf Bang and Jørn Dyerberg, confirmed this in studies between 1970 and 1979.[12] They found that the Greenlandic diet, which consists mainly of omega-3-rich seal and small whales, is similar to the Canadian Inuits' diet. The high consumption of polyunsaturated omega-3 fatty acids may explain the low incidence of cardiovascular diseases in these populations. It is true that the food in the diet of the Western world also includes polyunsaturated fatty acids, especially since vegetable margarine has replaced butter on most people's lunch tables; but these belong to another family—the omega-6 fatty acids. Let's define these further.

OMEGA-3 VERSUS OMEGA-6 FATTY ACIDS

As previously defined, the two largest categories of essential fatty acids are the omega-3 and omega-6 fatty acids. Omega-6 essential fatty acids help the body cure skin diseases, fight cancer cells, and treat arthritis. We need them in moderation, but most people consume an overabundance of this pro-inflammatory fat, which is found in meats, some vegetables, vegetable oils (vegetable oil is the number one source of fat in the American diet), legumes, nuts, and seeds.

Omega-3s are the fatty acids that deserve a halo because they serve a variety of important purposes within the body, as I've already been describing. To recap, they help your cells and organs to function properly, aid in the formation of cellular walls, and encourage the circulation of oxygen throughout the body. A lack of omega-3 essential fatty acids is known to lead to blood clots. If you seriously lack omega-3s, you might have problems with memory and mood, a decreased sense of vision, hair and skin issues, an irregular heartbeat, and a decrease in the functioning of your immune system. Mounting evidence also suggests that a high-fat diet rich in omega-3 fats prevents the development of insulin resistance more than does a diet high in saturated or omega-6 polyunsaturated fats. In liver cells, skeletal muscle, and fat cells, an omega-3-rich diet can increase the binding affinity of insulin to the insulin receptor, and in skeletal muscle and adipose tissue, an omega-3-rich diet increases tissue insulin sensitivity.

That's the good news. But here's the bad news: omega-3s are not as present in the standard American diet. The average American diet contains up to twenty times more omega-6s than omega-3s, and that is not a good thing. That means we're creating an imbalance in our bodies that ultimately prevents us from dialing up autophagy.

During Paleolithic times, the ratio of omega-6 to omega-3 fatty acids that humans ate varied from about 2 to 1 to 1 to 1. Modern US diets are about 20 to 1, down to maybe 10 to 1 for people who eat few processed foods. This is especially true of people who don't eat fish regularly or take enough supplemental omega-3 fish oil. More recent studies show that omega-6 fats increase hunger (and thus lead to obesity), whereas omega-3 fats decrease it. Going on a paleo diet will generally help balance this ratio, since doing away with processed foods, vegetable-based cooking oils, mayonnaise, and most nuts and eating low-glycemic carbs will greatly diminish the amount of that bad, inflammation-inducing oil in your diet. Although you'd think that eating meats and meat fats would help, the big difference has to do with what the animals those meats are from themselves ate.

Back in Paleolithic days, large game animals were all eating wild grasses and moving from place to place, so they generally didn't deplete the ground of minerals. Their own ratios of omega-6 to omega-3 fats was close to 2 to 1 and sometimes 1 to 1. So eating their fat was healthy. But in modern concentrated animal feeding operations (CAFOs), where thousands of cows, pigs, or chickens are penned up and not allowed to graze freely, the animals are generally fed nearly all grain, a majority of which is corn (and, as previously noted, sometimes soy and other supplements). A T-bone steak from a corn-fed cow has about 9 grams of saturated fat, whereas an equivalent piece from a purely grass-fed cow has about 1.3 grams.[13] Though the ratio of omega-6 to omega-3 is far better in grass-fed than grain-fed cattle, the total amount of omega-6 fats taken in by frequent consumption of beef is probably not going to significantly increase one's levels of inflammation, compared to the amounts of omega-6 consumed in vegetable oils (corn, soybean, and safflower, for example) and nuts. And since those oils are used in most processed foods, it's a largely unseen hazard.

Speaking of nuts, I want to point out something you've likely not heard about before. When you look closely at the list below, notice the surprisingly high omega-6 content of walnuts and almonds. We are often told that nuts contain "healthy fat," but I'd argue that, just like fats, not all nuts are created equal. The only nuts that pass my test to eat every day are macadamias, which have the best omega-3-to-omega-6 ratio, and in which most of the fats are monounsaturated. Almonds, peanuts (which are actually legumes), and Brazil nuts have essentially zero omega-3 fats and extremely high omega-6 levels. Don't get me wrong: Almonds, peanuts, walnuts, and Brazil nuts (among others) can be part of a healthy diet for sure, but if you're eating a lot of nuts on a daily basis, I'd opt for a kind that has a better ratio of omega-3 to omega-6 (and besides, if you're choosing between an omega-6 heavy processed food product and a handful of nuts, go for the nuts no matter what kind they are).

OMEGA-6 VERSUS OMEGA-3 CONTENT IN VARIOUS FOODS

Food	Calories	Omega-6	Omega-3	Saturated	N6/N3 Ratio
Tuna, canned in water, light, 1 can (165 g)	191	15	464	0	0.03
Shrimp, cooked, 16 large, 3 oz. (85 g)	84	18	295	0	0.06
Salmon, sockeye, dry-heat cooked, 3 oz. (85 g)	184	96	1210	2	0.08
Broccoli rabe, cooked, 3 oz. (85 g)	28	17	111	0	0.15
Spinach, raw, 2 cups (60 g)	14	16	83	0	0.19
Flaxseed, whole seeds, 1 tbsp. (10 g)	102	606	2338	400	0.26
Salmon, Atlantic, farmed, dry-heat cooked, 3 oz. (85 g)	175	566	1921	2	0.29
Romaine, 2 cups (85 g)	14	40	96	0	0.42
Broccoli, cooked, ½ cup (78 g)	27	40	93	0	0.43
Kidney beans, cooked, 1 cup (177 g)	225	191	301	0	0.63

Food	Calories	Omega-6	Omega-3	Saturated	N6/N3 Ratio
Kale, cooked, ½ cup (65 g)	18	52	67	0	0.78
Walnuts, 1 oz. (14 halves) (28 g)	185	10761	2565	1700	4.2
Peas, green, frozen, boiled, ½ cup (80 g)	62	84	19	0	4.42
Beef, grass-fed, ground, raw, 4 oz. (112 g)	216	480	100	6000	4.8
Soy oil, 2 tbsp., 1 oz. (28 g)	248	14361	1935	4	7.42
Soybeans, cooked, 1 cup (172 g)	298	7681	1029	2	7.46
Tofu, raw, firm, ½ cup (126 g)	183	5466	733	2	7.46
Chicken, breast meat only, roasted, diced, 1 cup (140 g)	231	826	98	1	8.43
Chicken, leg meat only, roasted, diced, 1 cup (140 g)	267	2268	238	3	9.53

Food	Calories	Omega-6	Omega-3	Saturated	N6/N3 Ratio
Beef, conventional, ground, raw, 4 oz. (112 g)	372	668	68	12800	9.82
Olive oil, 2 tbsp., 1 oz. (28 g)	248	2734	213	3900	12.84
McDonald's Chicken McNuggets, 4 pieces (64 g)	186	3505	191	2	18.35
Oatmeal, old-fashioned, regular, dry, $\frac{1}{3}$ cup (27 g)	102	594	27	300	22
Brown rice, medium grain, cooked, 1 cup (195 g)	218	552	25	0	22.08
Beef patty, pan-browned, 4 oz. (112 g)	304	452	20	8000	22.6
Corn, boiled, 1 large ear, 8 in. (118 g)	127	691	21	0	32.9
Peanut butter sandwich cookies (à la Girl Scout), 3 cookies (42 g)	201	1548	45	2	34.4
Corn oil, 2 tbsp., 1 oz. (28 g)	238	14448	314	3	46.01

Food	Calories	Omega-6	Omega-3	Saturated	N6/N3 Ratio
Pistachios, dry-roasted, 1 oz. (28 g)	160	3818	73	1600	52.3
Sesame seeds, raw, 2 tbsp. (18 g)	104	3848	68	1	56.59
Pumpkin seeds, 1 oz. (28 g)	153	5849	51	3	114.69
Peanut butter, 2 tbsp. (32 g)	188	3610	16	3000	225.63
Sunflower seeds, uncooked, 1 oz. (28 g)	164	6454	21	1200	307.33
Peanuts, Valencia, raw, 1 oz. (28 g)	160	4616	3	2100	1538.67
Almonds, blanched, 1 oz. (28 g)	161	3378	2	1000	1689

Key: Omega-6, the lower the better; omega-3, the higher the better; saturated fat, the lower the better; omega-6-to-omega-3 ratio, the lower the better

We've known for a long time that too many omega-6 fats can be hazardous to our health. In 1966, the Sydney Diet Heart Study, named after the Australian city in which it originated, randomly assigned 448 middle-aged men with a prior heart attack to either eat as they chose or eat a diet low in trans fats and cholesterol but rich in omega-6 fats (primarily safflower oil).[14] For seven years the researchers tracked the heart attacks and deaths in both groups. The results shocked everyone: despite a sharp drop in their LDL cholesterol levels, 6 percent more men died in the diet group, suggesting that 1 out of 18 had died *because of the diet*. Blood tests during the study showed that cholesterol and triglyceride levels dropped substantially in the diet group, precisely the intended effect. But the final outcome was a 6 percent increase in fatal heart problems—accounting completely for the difference in survival. The Sydney Diet, focused as it was on substituting bad fats (trans fats and dietary cholesterol) with omega-6 fatty acids, actually increased coronary and cardiac deaths!

The most powerful statement on the role of diet in preventing heart disease came more recently from the Lyon Diet Heart Study, which concluded in 1999.[15] In that study, survivors of heart attacks were split into two groups. One group was put on a diet that followed the American Heart Association recommendations (basically the USDA's guidelines, then called the Food Pyramid), and the second group was placed on a Mediterranean-type diet rich in fruits, vegetables, and fish. They also supplemented with omega-3 fatty acids and consumed very little omega-6s. At the end of four years, the two groups shared similar cholesterol levels. There was, however, a more than 70 percent reduction in both fatal and nonfatal heart attacks in the group on the Mediterranean diet compared with the AHA diet group, who were allowed to eat hefty amounts of omega-6 fatty acids.

That study poked holes in the high-cholesterol theory of heart disease. In fact, the study was terminated early due to the significant benefits found in the group on the Mediterranean diet compared to the other group. More important, during the four years the group was on the Mediterranean diet, they experienced no sudden cardiac deaths (a term used to describe electrical chaos in the heart, which makes it stop beating in rhythm and is the primary cause of cardiovascular-related death). The researchers also documented more new cancers in the AHA diet group than in the Mediterranean diet group. There were no significant differences between the two groups in terms of tobacco use, medications used (including antilipids), exercise, weight, blood pressure, and psychosocial factors. This allowed the scientists to home in on the effects of just their nutrient intake.

Clearly, the American Heart Association's pronouncements can be imperfect. In 2017, the AHA published a statement condemning coconut oil, calling it an unhealthy saturated fat.[16] It stirred an uproar in the medical community because the statement created confusion. Some critics called out the AHA's relationship with a donor that was also a producer of soybeans, suspicious that a financial incentive was behind the recommendation. The current consensus is that coconut oil is not "unhealthy" when it is consumed in its pure and natural form—not in combination with refined grains. It can be a great cooking oil and a flavorful addition to dishes, as well as a source of those medium-chain triglycerides. I don't think anyone is going to overdose on coconut oil.

HAIL TO OMEGA-3S!

Omega-3 fats speed up metabolism (animals such as sea birds and seals that eat an omega-3-rich diet have unusually high metabolisms given their body size) and help shut down inflammation in the body, whereas omega-6 fats slow metabolism down and ramp up inflammation. This may be one key to why the modern diet makes us fat and prone to chronic illness rooted in inflammation. It's not just that we're eating too much food, it's that we're also eating a diet dominated by omega-6s. Having a high omega-6-to-omega-3 ratio can be bad for your bones, too, as a higher ratio has been linked with lower bone mineral density.

Omega-6 comes from many seeds and grains and is particularly high in the kinds of vegetable oils we rely on in the Western world. The most common oil in processed food—soybean oil—is almost 90 percent omega-6s. Soybean oil is currently the biggest source of omega-6 fatty acids in the United States because it is really cheap (the amount of omega-6 fatty acids found in our body fat stores has increased by more than 200 percent, or threefold, in the past fifty years alone). And this isn't just because we changed our diet; we also changed the diet of the animals we eat. We're increasingly feeding them omega-6-rich grain (corn is high in omega-6s) rather than wild plants and grasses, thereby dramatically reducing the omega-3 content of most CAFO meats.

HEALTHY FATS IN THE MEDITERRANEAN DIET

The term "Mediterranean diet," implying that all Mediterranean people follow the same diet, is a misnomer. The countries around the Mediterranean Basin—in the region of lands around the Mediterranean Sea—have different diets, religions, and cultures. Their diets differ in the quality of fat consumption, type of meat, and volume of wine intake; the use of milk versus cheese; the variety of fruits and vegetables; and the rates of coronary heart disease and cancer. Greece has the lowest disease rates and longest life expectancy in the area. Extensive studies on the traditional diet of Greece (the diet before Western influences crept onto the scene starting in 1960) indicate that the dietary pattern of Greeks consists of a higher intake of fruits, vegetables (particularly wild plants), nuts, and grains (mostly in the form of low-glycemic sourdough bread rather than high-glycemic pasta); more olive oil and olives; less cow's milk but more goat's milk and sheep's milk cheeses; more fish; less meat; and less wine than those in other Mediterranean countries.

Analysis of the dietary pattern of the residents of Crete shows a number of protective substances, such as selenium, glutathione, a balanced ratio of omega-6 to omega-3 essential fatty acids, high amounts of fiber, antioxidants (especially resveratrol from wine and polyphenols from olive oil), and vitamins E and C, some of which have been shown to be associated with lower risk of cancer, including cancer of the breast.[17] So when I endorse a "Mediterranean diet," I'm really talking about a traditional Greek diet. It's the best diet for leveraging the power of autophagy and its antidisease processes.

In April 2013, *The New England Journal of Medicine* published a large landmark study showing that people aged 55 to 80 who ate a Mediterranean diet were at lower risk of developing heart disease and stroke than those on a typical low-fat diet.[18] The reduction was shown to be as much as 30 percent. The results were so alarming that the researchers halted the study early because the low-fat diet proved too damaging for the people eating lots of commercially baked goods rather than sources of healthy fats. (In 2018, the authors of that study retracted their original paper and republished a reanalysis of their data in the same journal following criticism of their methodology.[19] Although there were flaws in the original study, mainly due to the limitations of conducting studies on diet outcomes and controlling for factors the researchers couldn't really control, the conclusion remained the same.)

The Mediterranean-style diet also got the spotlight in 2017 for its apparent support of brain health—specifically brain volume. The brain tends to atrophy with age, so anything to keep its volume (and strength) is a bonus. That year, a study was published in the journal *Neurology* showing that older people who adhered closely to the diet had greater brain volume.[20] The Scottish researchers measured brain volume using magnetic resonance imaging of 401 people when they were 73 years old and again when they were 76. Even after adjusting for other factors that could explain the difference in brain volume, such as diabetes, hypertension, and even education, the researchers' conclusions were clear: lower adherence to a Mediterranean-style diet is predictive of brain atrophy over a three-year period. Interestingly, the participants with the strongest adherence averaged 10 milliliters greater total brain volume than those with the lowest.

There's plenty of research to show the positive effects of a

Mediterranean diet on type 2 diabetes as well. When researchers reviewed multiple studies in this area, their conclusion was that the evidence so far accumulated suggests that adopting a Mediterranean diet may help prevent the onset of type 2 diabetes and improve glycemic control and lower cardiovascular risk in persons who already have diabetes.[21] Several of the reported studies showed improvement of fasting glucose and hemoglobin A1c (blood sugar) levels in those on the Mediterranean diet, as well as fewer cardiovascular events.

The possibility of an increased likelihood of stroke has been raised by numerous researchers studying high-dose fish oils. This is because the epidemiological data regarding Greenland Eskimos indicated that they seemed to have higher stroke rates than did Danes. This potential side effect of high-dose fish oil was addressed by studies that compared Japanese fishing villages and farming communities located twenty miles apart.[22] The researchers found a much lower incidence of stroke in the fishing villages (where people consumed more fish) than among the farmers (who consumed much less fish and therefore less fish oil). The residents of the fishing villages had an omega-6-to-omega-3 ratio of 1.5 to 1 in their blood, the lower limit that I recommend (see chapter 9). In another study, Greenland Eskimos who had suffered a hemorrhagic stroke had an omega-6-to-omega-3 ratio of 0.5 to 1, a third of the lower limit that I recommend, while those who had not suffered a stroke had an omega-6 to omega-3 ratio of 0.8 to 1, which is still only half of the lower limit that I recommend.[23] If the omega-6-to-omega-3 ratio is a third of my recommendation, there might be an increased risk of stroke. However, due to the high amounts of omega-6 fats Americans generally consume, even Alzheimer's disease patients taking 25 grams of long-chain omega-3 fatty acids each day rarely had their omega-6 to omega-3 ratio drop below 1.5 to 1.

Another way to circumvent this potential problem is to use extra-virgin olive oil whenever possible. Extra-virgin olive oil is exceptionally rich in antioxidants compared with other mono-unsaturated oils, since it is derived from a fruit (the olive) rather than a seed. Olive oil contains a very potent antioxidant called squalene that has been shown to virtually eliminate any increase in oxidation products in the bloodstream that may occur with high-dose fish oil. That's why monounsaturated fats, especially olive oil, are a major constituent of my dietary plan.

Of course, taking 100 to 400 IU of vitamin E per day as a supplement is another way to circumvent this potential problem. You can easily have your ratio tested with kits available online. A ratio between 1.5 to 1 and 3 to 1 indicates that your "good" and "bad" omegas are in balance and that you are in the omega zone of wellness. In the program outlined in chapter 9, I'll give you some suggestions for making sure you're getting your omegas right. If you do not want to consume foods that will deliver these nutri-ents, supplementation will be key.

Though numerous studies have shown specific benefits from supplementing with omega-3 fatty acids, a prestigious 2018 study published in Cochran Database of Systematic Reviews found that a review of seventy-nine clinical studies involving omega-3 supplementation resulted in no reduction in all-mortality or heart disease–related deaths in the treated subjects.[24] Looking through the cited studies, I noted that they generally used far lower doses of omega-3s than I believe are necessary (and an order of magnitude less than levels consumed by peoples near the Arctic Circle, who enjoy an omega-3-rich diet). I've come to believe that one must approach a cellular membrane level of omega-3 fatty acids in the 8 percent range on the omega-3 index blood test. By consuming one tablespoon a day of liquid (flavored) fish oil, I was able to get my level up to about 10 percent in just a few months, as measured by this commercially available blood test.

It's difficult to overdose on omega-3s, which will ultimately help you gravitate toward foods that will power up your body's autophagy forces.

Top Sources of Omega-3 Fatty Acids

Dark green leafy vegetables (e.g., broccoli, salad greens)

Cold-water fatty wild fish (e.g., salmon, mackerel)

Pasture-raised (grass-fed) meat

Pastured eggs

Hempseed

Flaxseed

Chia seeds

Extra-virgin olive oil

Coconut oil

Avocado oil

Macadamia nuts

Fish oil

Vegan-friendly supplements containing EPA and DHA
from algae

Deep-Six the Omega-6 Fatty Acids

Vegetable oils high in omega-6 (sunflower, corn, soybean, peanut, and cottonseed)

Processed foods that contain these oils

Many legumes, nuts, and seeds

CHAPTER 8

WHALES, RODENTS, AND SMOKERS

Just as Laron syndrome dwarfs showed us how reduced IGF-1 can result in cancer resistance, we can learn other lessons from some distant mammalian cousins about suppressing that disease by periodically turning down the mTOR switch and thus turning up autophagy. Cancer is, after all, one of the most feared ailments. Among all the causes of human death, natural or man-made, cancer stands at number two (after heart disease). That's about 1 in every 4 deaths. Turns out that bowhead whales, naked mole rats, and even light smokers can demonstrate ways to turn down mTOR to avoid this malady. Their habits further point to the power of autophagy.

Though it may seem odd to study the habits and environment of whales, rodents, and smokers in the hope of improving human health, this is how science is often conducted. We learn wherever we can.

MEET THE BOWHEAD WHALE

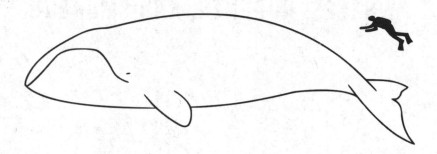

Bowhead whales aren't the largest mammals in the sea, but they have the largest mouths of any living animals, taking up one-third of their entire body length. They can grow up to 65 feet long, with extremely large heads and relatively stocky (short and fat) bodies. They also have the thickest blubber of any animal, which unfortunately made them a prized target of whalers, who over the past several hundred years have decimated their numbers. The whales live in the Northern Hemisphere, around the pack ice of the polar regions, often in shallow waters. Unlike other whales, they do not migrate to warmer waters, staying in the freezing waters above the Arctic Circle, though they move to other areas within the Arctic waters between summer feeding areas and wintering areas. These whales are baleen whales, which means they have plates of whalebone in their mouth, and they filter their food through their long baleen bristles. Bowhead whales open their giant mouths and graze along the surface or on the sea floor, scooping up zooplankton, including copepods and euphausiids. They need to eat about 100 metric tons of crustaceans per year. Their food is very rich in omega-3 fatty acids, and as a result, not surprisingly, bowhead blubber contains relatively high levels of omega-3 fatty acids and no detectable omega-6 fatty acids. It's also very high in vitamin D as a result of their diet.

From the seventeenth through the early twentieth centuries, bowhead whales were commercially hunted for oil, meat, and apparel materials (corset stays, umbrella ribs, buggy whips, and more).[1] Today some Native Alaskans are allowed to hunt a limited number of bowhead whales for food and products to produce native handicrafts. Bowheads are also preyed upon by killer whales. Some die after becoming trapped and frozen in heavy ice, while others die of other natural causes. Their limited population and harsh aquatic home make bowheads the most difficult of all large whales to study. Because of their absence of teeth (which can be used to estimate age in other mammals), it is difficult to tell how old bowheads are when they die naturally. But we do have some clues to how long they can live if they are not killed by prey.

Dr. Craig George, senior wildlife biologist at the Department of Wildlife Management in Barrow, Alaska, utilized a technique to measure the age of bowhead whales by studying changes in the amino acids in the lenses of their eyes. In 2004, Dr. George and colleagues published an update on their age estimation of bowhead whales after studying forty-eight of the whales caught by Alaskan Eskimos (Inupiat) between 1978 and 1997.[2] To his astonishment, he found one that was 174 years old and another that was 213 years old! Bowhead whales are thus considered to be the longest-lived mammals on the planet.

The Inupiat have hunted whales for more than four thousand years with harpoons and often told of whales that several generations of hunters recognized by their markings, which occur on the skin of the whale when it pushes up against ice packs to break through. Those marks make them readily identifiable to a trained whaler. They are akin to an identifying tattoo.

The age estimates were supported by native hunters in Barrow and other villages along the frozen north coast of Alaska, who have found six ancient harpoon points in the blubber of freshly killed bowhead whales since 1981. These harpoon points were not made like modern-day ones, which are made of steel. The ones found in the bowheads were made of ivory and stone, which haven't been used since the 1880s.

According to many research reports, cancer is highly unusual among whales, dolphins, and porpoises. Among more than 1,800 cetaceans examined in the Canadian Arctic, only a single cancer was found, and no tumors were identified in approximately 50 belugas. Of 130 dead bowhead whales examined between 1980 and 1989, only one had a benign tumor, located in the liver. According to L. Michael Philo, writing about the causes of death in bowhead whales in the book *The Bowhead Whale*, "It is unlikely that tumors are major contributors to Bowhead whale morbidity or mortality."[3]

So what are the bowheads' longevity and anticancer secrets? Whereas their feeding is adequate during the summer, it is generally sparse during the dark, frigid winter months. During that time, they undergo extreme calorie restriction in which most of their nutrients come from ketogenesis and autophagy of their stored fat. This kind of pattern—keeping the Switch on nine months of the year, then having three months off—is one I'll endorse in my program. The story of the bowhead whale reiterates the value of intermittent seasonal fasting and calorie restriction (as the Mount Athos monks do) and following a ketogenic diet once in a while. But it also conveys the importance of letting the Switch turn up mTOR for certain periods of the year in order to build reserves and foster the growth of new tissues and cells.

Whales such as the bowhead add another twist to the mTOR story. They take deep dives and often hold their breath for twenty minutes to an hour, during which it is thought that they undergo intermittent hypoxia (oxygen deficiency). This is important since upstream of the mTOR switch are sensors not just for insulin and IGF-1, as well as adequate supplies of certain amino acids, such as leucine, but also for oxygen. Oxygen is critical to the energy-producing processes of cells, and because making proteins or dividing so as to produce a new daughter cell takes lots of energy, a cell will turn energy production down through mTOR if the oxygen levels aren't adequate. But bowhead whales aren't the only mammals to undergo intermittent fasting and hypoxia. The next species we will meet has an oily skin and large buckteeth.

THE NAKED MOLE RAT

Perhaps the phrase "a face only a mother could love" came while gazing at a naked mole rat, which has become a darling in scientific circles, though you probably wouldn't call it that at first glance.

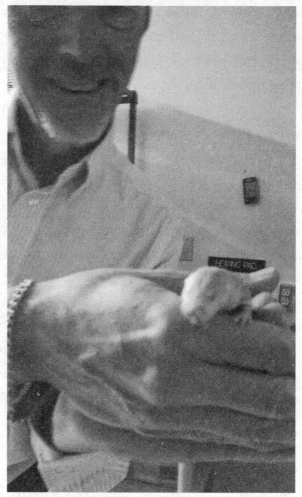

Me holding a naked mole rat

These rodents have hairless, tubular, wrinkled bodies with two large buckteeth that make them look a little like tiny walruses. And they are the only cold-blooded mammal on Earth, living in communities underground mostly in the desert regions of eastern Africa and the Middle East. I was allowed to hold one in my hands in the subterranean vivarium of Shelley Buffenstein, a professor at the Barshop Institute for Aging and Longevity Studies (a part of the University of Texas at San Antonio) and now a senior principal investigator at Calico Labs (a Google subsidiary), whose long-lived rodents are the focus of her research.

A colony can have anywhere from twenty to three hundred naked mole rats living in an underground area that can be as large as six football fields and have an elaborate tunnel system. Each member of a naked mole rat pack is assigned a different role. Some burrow tunnels; others gather roots and bulbs for the colony to eat. Other rats tend to the queen, who is the only one in the colony to breed. Male naked mole rats vie for hierarchy in the pecking order, and there's constantly a contest—males among males and females among females—as to who gets to be on top and who gets walked on in their cramped tunnels and rooms. They very rarely venture aboveground, and when they do it's usually in search of food; therefore they have to contend with far fewer predators than do aboveground rodents.

Unlike their rodent cousins mice and rats, who generally live two to five years at most, a naked mole rat can live as long as thirty years, showing no sign of aging until it's a quarter of a century old. Blind and plump, it skitters around in a hazmat suit of its own creation. And these rats' preferred living quarters are less than desirable by human standards. They love sleeping in piles of other naked mole rats, which, due to poor ventilation of their burrows, result in levels of gas, including carbon dioxide, that would kill other animals. The air in naked mole rat burrows is usually low in oxygen (approximately 8 percent) and high in carbon dioxide (approximately 10 percent) because of the poor gas exchange through the soil and because many naked mole rats share the same limited air supply. Therefore these animals live in a chronically hypoxic (low-oxygen) environment but are remarkably resistant to the negative effects of hypoxia. In nature, naked mole rats are restricted from foraging during dry seasons. They cannot search extensively for new food sources unless the ground has been sufficiently moistened by rain. During brief periods after rain, naked mole rats get to work, digging intensely to find enough food to sustain them through long droughts. Such a foraging pattern may keep them in a state of intermittent calorie restriction and lengthy fasting, which, as we've seen in previous chapters, induces autophagy, slows aging, and lengthens life span.

Naked mole rats maintain normal activity and body composition for at least 80 percent of their lives and have no obvious age-related increases in morbidity or mortality rate, despite their harsh living conditions. Their long life span may be attributed to sustained good health and a pronounced resistance to cancer. As you probably know, mice and rats are routinely used in research circles to study disease. Scientists give them all kinds of illnesses to study common ailments that affect humans; they also conduct interventional studies on rodents to see whether *x*, *y*, or *z* has any effect on their health (and in turn perhaps human health). In other words, most biomedical researchers want to make animals sick so they can try to find a cure. But here's the incredible thing about naked mole rats: you can't give them cancer. When Professor Buffenstein tried to induce cancer in them by infecting them, injecting them, or irradiating them, they didn't develop cancer. To the contrary, they *cured* themselves.

A few cases in point[4]: In 2004, she put some of these cancer-resistant rodents into a gamma radiation chamber and shot them with ionizing rays. None of their cells became cancerous. In 2010, she tried using a well-known cancer-causing virus and cancer-causing genes (SV40 TAg and Ras), but again the rats remained healthy. A year later, her lab attempted to give naked mole rats cancer by combining DMBA, a vicious carcinogen, and an inflammatory agent known as TPA. This combination kills 100 percent of the mice it's given to, but the naked mole rats refused to yield.

Naked mole rats have several mechanisms in place to ensure the health of their protein structures and homeostasis. Their proteins seem to be resistant to unfolding stressors such as high temperatures and urea (a nitrogenous breakdown product of metabolism), and their cells are particularly efficient at removing damaged proteins and organelles via what's called the ubiquitin-proteasome system and, you guessed it, autophagy. The ubiquitin-proteasome system is a long technical term that has a simple definition: it's basically a means of breaking down potentially harmful proteins that could foment cancer. Indeed, naked mole rat proteasomes both are more abundant and show greater efficiency in destroying stress-damaged proteins in liver tissue than do the proteasomes within the liver tissues of regular laboratory mice. Similarly, autophagy occurs at a two- to fourfold greater rate in naked mole rat cells than in mice or other rats.

This was confirmed by Shanmin Zhao, a scientist at the Second Military Medical University in Shanghai, China, who demonstrated in 2014 that naked mole rats have higher levels of autophagy than do laboratory mice.[5] Collectively, their enhanced intracellular cleaning processes may contribute to the better maintenance of a high-quality proteome and help the naked mole rat's cells resist damage when encountering cellular toxins, such as heavy metals or direct DNA-damaging agents. (Briefly, your proteome is the entire library of proteins that can be expressed by your body's cells and tissues; understanding how proteins become damaged is part of understanding how cancer develops.) It takes much higher concentrations of these toxins to kill naked mole rat cells than are needed to kill mouse cells subjected to the identical experimental treatment.

One other bizarre characteristic to note is that naked mole rats are impervious to certain forms of pain, such as the pain caused by eating fiery hot chili peppers and acids from lemon juice and vinegar. They have the ability to turn those harsh stimulants into analgesics. Research is under way today to see whether we might be able to make the human pain system similarly immune to this type of pain, which could be extremely helpful for patients with cancer or arthritis, for whom the buildup of acid in body tissue can be a major contributor to their chronic pain.

What can we take away from the naked mole rat's success in life? Is anything about its lifestyle applicable to us? Well, I've already called out the intermittent calorie restriction that no doubt helps spur their autophagy. But there's something else we can glean from the naked mole rat's oxygen-deprived living environment, which brings us to the potential benefits of light smoking.

SMOKE THIS

Jeanne Louise Calment was born in the town of Arles in southern France. In 1988, upon the centenary of Vincent van Gogh's visit to Arles, she told reporters that she had met the painter a hundred years previously, in 1888, as a thirteen-year-old girl in her uncle's fabric shop, when he wanted to buy some canvas, later describing him as "dirty, badly dressed and disagreeable" and "very ugly, ungracious, impolite, sick." Her personal knowledge of van Gogh led her to having a part, playing herself, in the 1990 film *Vincent et Moi*.

Jeanne Louise is best remembered for the fact that she's verified to be the oldest woman to have ever lived. She died in August 1997 in Arles at the age of 122 years and 164 days.[*] One or more books about her and a documentary film about her life, *Beyond 120 Years with Jeanne Calment*, have also come out. Like many individuals who live to an exceptional age, she did not lead a pristine, healthy life. She spent her days doing almost everything that doctors advise against if you want to live long. She smoked, she drank—allowing herself one glass of port and one cigarette a day. She played with guns, she ate excessive amounts of sugar and red meat, and she never ate breakfast, save for a cup or two of coffee. She started smoking when she was 16 and quit (upon the insistence of her doctor) at age 116—smoking for a hundred years straight. Two of the world's longest-lived men, Christian Mortensen, who lived for 115

---

[*]Jeanne's age has been certified by the Guinness World Records and public researchers, but some have accused her of lying about her age. It still stands in the record books, and challenges to her age have been called ridiculous.

years and 252 days, and Walter Breuning, who lived for 114 years and 205 days, smoked cigars daily until their early 100s. (And we all remember George Burns and his famous cigar smoking; he lived to 100.)

Clearly, Jeanne Louise is the exception, not the rule. But her story brings up two important points. Note that I said she didn't eat breakfast save for coffee. That means she fasted every night and started her day with a pro-autophagy drink (yes, coffee stimulates autophagy through its polyphenol content; polyphenols are a group of more than five hundred phytochemicals, which are naturally occurring micronutrients in plants that give a plant its color and can help protect it from various dangers). Now, is it possible that her daily cigarette helped her, too? Let me be clear: I am not going to endorse smoking of any kind. Let's get that straight. But I do want to point out some interesting chemistry here so you don't panic the next time you inhale something that competes with your oxygen.

Cigarettes produce a small amount of carbon monoxide. This gas will fit so strongly into the oxygen-binding pocket of hemoglobin (the oxygen-carrying protein in our red blood cells) that it cannot be released again. In the competition between oxygen and carbon monoxide, carbon monoxide is the clear winner. Some gas heaters are so efficient at taking CO_2 (carbon dioxide) and turning it into CO (carbon monoxide) that building codes require the installation of carbon monoxide sensor alarms to warn of high CO levels so that occupants won't suffocate. Thus, inhaling carbon monoxide from cigarettes can temporarily cause mild hypoxia. There is something to be said for starving cells of oxygen under the right conditions. Both bowhead whales and naked mole rats frequently endure hypoxia, which may account for their increased state of activation of autophagy.

Although it's possible that the transient hypoxia induced by smoking a single cigarette or enjoying the smoke of a cigar once a day could actually turn on autophagy and thus help rid the alveoli of damaged proteins, exogenous particles, and malfunctioning organelles, it could also be the case that supercentenarians simply have one or more protective genes that provide them with an adequate defense against the harmful effects of inhaling tobacco, which would likely be absent from others who attempt to practice the same habit. So again, I am not endorsing smoking, but the conversation is too intriguing to omit when trying to fully understand autophagy across species. It also allows me to transition to the topic of hormesis: When is a substance that's toxic at high doses actually *protective* at low doses?

THE POWER OF POISON

Mithradates (Mith-ruh-*dayt*-ees) is a Persian name, generally associated with the royal family that ruled an ancient kingdom of Pontus in what is now northeast Turkey. King Mithradates V was part Greek (claiming lineage from Alexander the Great) and part Persian (the son of King Pharnaces I of Pontus). He was a friend of Rome and supplied it with ships and soldiers during the Third Punic War, in which Rome fought the Carthaginians. About thirty years into his reign, King Mithradates was assassinated by poison, possibly on orders from his wife, the queen. Mithradates VI, the eldest son of the king and queen, fearing that his mother might try to poison him, too, in order to give the throne to her favored son, began ingesting nonlethal amounts of poisons, and later, after hundreds of experiments, created a mixture of poisons that he thought would make him immune to all known poisons.

Mithradates VI was no friend of Rome, however, and fought fierce battles against the republic throughout his life. After his death (by suicide), the "Poison King's" secret formula was imbibed by kings and queens, royalty, and others as far away as China in a practice called mithridatism, i.e., protecting oneself against poisoning by taking small amounts of poisons.

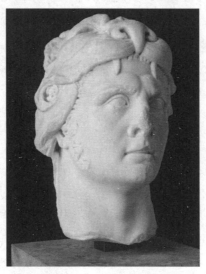

Bust of Mithradates VI at the Louvre, Paris, France

In the past few decades, scientists have begun to discover a "counterintuitive" process having properties quite like Mithradates' antidote, called hormesis. (This is not to be confused with homeopathy. Generalizations of the hormesis phenomenon used in support of homeopathy are unfounded.)

Hormesis is described as a dose-response relationship phenomenon characterized by low-dose stimulation and high-dose inhibition. That is, the agent in question has a biphasic curve (a U curve) in which a low dose will stimulate an effect ranging from 30 to 60 percent over the effect with no dose at all and a much higher dose will inhibit the response.[6] Confusing? An example will help illustrate: A particular chemotherapy drug may stimulate tumor growth at low doses but inhibit it at higher doses. Thus, from a tumor cell's viewpoint, a small dose of this chemotherapy toxin is healthful and stimulates it to grow, whereas more of it will cause it to die. As the scientists describe this new concept—remarkably akin to Mithradates' own hypothesis—minute doses of poisonous substances can be beneficial, analogous to a vaccine. It is well documented, for another example, that drinking moderate amounts of alcohol (not just wine but any alcoholic beverage) lowers the risk of heart disease, whereas higher consumption is associated with higher risks of developing heart and liver disease, neurological disorders, and cancer.[7] Other studies indicate that low doses of many chemical toxins, whether from smog, cadmium, pesticides, or dioxin, appear to have hormetic effects.[8] But again, it's all about the dose (and don't get me wrong: I'm *not* suggesting you add a splash of pesticide to your morning coffee).

Let me give you one more easy example so you can nail this concept: Scientists have long documented that vigorous aerobic exercise extends life span in animals and reduces a myriad of age-related diseases in humans (and the exercise needn't necessarily be vigorous all the time to reap the benefits). But there's a paradox here because aerobic exercise is toxic to the body to some degree. It's *aerobic*, meaning it involves high-volume oxygen throughput, up to ten times the rate when the body is at rest. In response to such exercise, cells fortify themselves by increasing the expression of genes involved in oxygen defense and cellular repair. This is the essence of hormesis.

The researcher in the United States who has been most responsible for helping turn around the scientific opinion about the role of small doses of toxins in good health is Edward Calabrese, a toxicologist and professor in the School of Public Health and Health Sciences at the University of Massachusetts Amherst. His interest sprang from an experiment he performed as an undergraduate student at Bridgewater State College in 1966. In the experiment, he and his classmates sprayed a peppermint plant with a common herbicide called Phosfon (chlorphonium chloride), planning to measure how much it stunted the plant's growth. But much to their surprise, the plant responded by growing approximately 40 percent taller and leafier than untreated plants did. Later, they discovered that the herbicide had accidentally been diluted too much. That accident jolted Calabrese's curiosity, and he went on to study a paradox in toxicology that had been around for a long time but hadn't seen much daylight: whether low doses of some poisons could actually be beneficial.

In 1998, after spending nearly a decade gathering data from thousands of studies, Calabrese published a paper showing that chemical hormesis was likely to have occurred in 350 of the nearly 4,000 studies he evaluated.[9] Numerous biological endpoints were assessed; growth responses were the most prevalent, followed by metabolic effects, longevity, reproductive responses, and survival. He found instances where bacteria thrived in minute doses of antibiotics; plants exploded in growth after being given tiny doses of heavy metals such as lead; and rats exposed to a little DDT had fewer liver tumors than unexposed rats. His conclusion was that chemical hormesis is a reproducible and relatively common biological phenomenon. The theory does have its critics and it's currently under study around the world, but the underlying mechanism seems logical: when an organism is faced with a potential threat to survival, it will respond by unleashing biological processes and molecular repair crews. That reaction could in effect benefit the organism in some way.* And here's where autophagy may come into play.

XENOPHAGY: SELF-EATING THE "STRANGERS WITHIN"

First, some more biology will help. White blood cells, also known as leukocytes (from the Greek words *leuko*, meaning "white," and

---

*One of the most interesting areas of study today regarding the potential power of hormesis revolves around the use of "buckyballs," which are nanoparticles of carbon molecules that form a spherical shape resembling a soccer ball. They have been shown to have antioxidant properties that may ultimately promote autophagy and extend life. They also may work by stressing the cells via hormesis. One 2017 study that went viral over the internet came from France, where researchers injected rats' stomachs with buckyballs dissolved in olive oil and the rats lived twice as long. This kind of research has its skeptics, but it's only in its infancy, so there's no practical takeaway for us yet. But stay tuned. Maybe one day we'll all be drinking buckyballs in our morning coffee. In 1985, Robert Curl and Richard Smalley at Rice University in Houston, and Harold Kroto at the University of Sussex in the United Kingdom, created the hollow, spherical carbon clusters. They were named Buckminsterfullerenes (later just "fullerenes" or "buckyballs"), in honor of the noted futurist and inventor Buckminster Fuller, who had designed a geodesic dome that looked very similar in structure. In 1996, the three scientists won the Nobel Prize in Chemistry for their work.

kytos, meaning "hollow vessel"), are immune system cells made in our bone marrow by stem cells. They are found throughout the body, including in the blood and the lymphatic system. An uncommonly high number of white blood cells in the blood is generally an indicator of disease. Macrophages (from the Greek for "big eaters") are a type of white blood cell that engulf and digest cellular debris outside the cells. Their targets include cellular debris, as when a cell dies and decomposes, foreign substances, microbes, and rogue cells, such as cancer cells. They can be inflammatory by releasing nitric oxide, or they can be reparative by releasing a growth hormone molecule, ornithine.

Another extracellular protector is the phagocytes (from the Greek *phagein*, meaning "to eat," and *cyte*, meaning "cell"). These are cells that protect the body by ingesting harmful foreign particles, bacteria, and dead or dying cells. Phagocytes are attracted to invaders by chemical signals that are given off during an infection. When they come into contact with, say, bad bacteria, they engulf it and kill it with oxidants or nitric oxide. A cell membrane will form a vesicle around a particle that has been absorbed by a phagocyte. This vesicle is called a phagosome, and it will then fuse with a lysosome to digest the foreign invader. These terms should sound familiar, because phagosomes and lysosomes play key roles in digesting or recycling biological components in the autophagy process I described in chapter 2.

Sadly for multicellular organisms like us, bacteria have had a long time to gain skill at evading these systems and making it into cells, where they try to hijack the cellular equipment so as to infect their host and proliferate. Antibacterial autophagy, also known as xenophagy (from Greek meaning "stranger" or "foreigner" plus "eating"), is an innate component of the immune response, which is directed against intracellular pathogens, such as viruses and bacteria.

Ubiquitin, first identified in 1975, is a small regulatory protein that is present in nearly all cells (hence from "ubiquitous") that have nuclei (they are not found in red blood cells). These proteins bind to other proteins that need to be digested via autophagy. The target proteins can be singular (by themselves), bound to other proteins, or part of a bacterium or virus. Of course, some bacteria have evolved to evade the xenophagy, too. Salmonella, for instance, can block autophagic defenses in later stages of its infectious cycle, whereas HIV contains a protein called Nef that appears to block autophagosome maturation. When Nef is blocked, the HIV virus is degraded by the xenophagy process.

Now let's bring this discussion back to the notion of a toxin being a stimulator of autophagy. The cleaning process can be triggered by the sensing of toxins within the cell and mitochondria. It is believed that autophagy of particular viruses, bacteria, and parasites can be considered, at least in part, to be a reaction to the physical properties of these objects rather than a response to their chemical structure and/or the products of their metabolism, but the exact method by which they're identified is still not known. Mutated or damaged mitochondria can give off higher levels of free radicals than healthy mitochondria do, and these dysfunctional powerhouses can also be tagged for removal by autophagy. Taking antioxidant supplements may reduce free radicals (also more technically called reactive oxygen species, or ROS) that signals that the mitochondria should be recycled and thus interfere with getting rid of dysfunctional mitochondria. This may explain a paradox that has haunted researchers trying to solve health problems by increasing the body's supply of antioxidants. (Among the body's own antioxidants naturally produced are alpha lipoic acid and glutathione.)

REVERSE HORMESIS

We constantly hear about the benefits of antioxidants. They are in the daily media and are touted as antiaging gems in products from those we put on our face to the food we ingest. Technically, antioxidants include vitamins, carotenes, phytochemicals, and minerals found in food and plants. They act as electron donors to quench free radicals that are capable of damaging proteins, cell membranes, and our DNA. As a result, they can potentially lead to inflammation and an increased risk of developing cancer and many chronic diseases. But if you've been paying attention to those same media, you may have noticed a few years back when headlines such as "Antioxidants CAUSE Cancer!" made waves. After decades of research examining the potential benefits of consuming antioxidants or rubbing them into our skin, what brought about that alarming news story?

Several clinical trials worldwide have been done on antioxidant supplementation and cancer prevention. The results, however, have not been totally clear. In most cases, supplementation has been shown to have no impact on the risk for a variety of cancers. But we cannot ignore the studies that have demonstrated an *increased* cancer risk. The most notable of these studies were the Carotene and Retinol Efficacy Trial (CARET)[10] and the Alpha-

Tocopherol, Beta-Carotene Cancer Prevention (ATBC) study[11] in which daily supplementation with beta-carotene or a combination of beta-carotene and vitamin A increased lung cancer incidence and all-cause mortality in smokers. Both studies began in 1985; the CARET study was halted in early 1996 ahead of schedule due to the alarming results. People taking the supplements in the ATBC study did so until 1993 but were followed until 2013. There was also the Selenium and Vitamin E Cancer Prevention Trial (SELECT), which initially published its results in 2008[12] with a follow-up in 2011[13]; SELECT showed that daily vitamin E supplementation increased prostate cancer in older men by as much as 17 percent.

In a 2015 study, University of Gothenburg scientists gave vitamin E and a generic drug called N-acetylcysteine (N-A-C or NAC), both antioxidants, to mice with early-stage lung cancer.[14] The vitamin E doses were comparable to those in supplements. The doses of acetylcysteine, which is prescribed for chronic obstructive pulmonary disease (COPD) to reduce mucus production, were relatively low. The results were eye-opening: the antioxidants caused a 2.8-fold increase in lung tumors compared to mice not given antioxidants. Moreover, the antioxidants apparently made the tumors more invasive and aggressive, causing the mice to die twice as quickly as the antioxidant-free mice. And when the antioxidants were added to human lung tumor cells in lab dishes, they also accelerated their growth. That result agreed with the many studies finding that "antioxidants do not protect against cancer in healthy people and may increase it" or promote it in those who already do have cancer. That's according to Martin Bergö, who led the 2015 study. Bergö was also involved in another

2015 study that showed antioxidants increasing the risk of skin cancer (melanoma) becoming metastatic.[15]

The significant advance in Bergö's lung study was pinpointing how antioxidants can be, counterintuitively, pro-cancer. Antioxidants do indeed decrease oxidative stress and DNA damage, as expected. But the damage becomes so insignificant as to be undetectable by the cell. And when that happens, the cell fails to deploy its cancer defense system, which is based on a protein called p53. This anticancer molecule and the tumor-suppressing gene that encodes it—TP53—has gotten a lot of attention in the past thirty-odd years, especially since *Science* magazine declared it "Molecule of the Year" in December 1993.* It's the most popular gene studied today. (On average, around two papers are published each day describing new details of the basic biology of TP53.) Here's the thing: it is mutated in roughly half of all human cancers. Here's the other thing: we humans have only a single copy of it per set of chromosomes, which calculates to two copies per cell—one from Mom and another from Dad. Lots of other animals that evade cancer entirely have more copies of TP53. Elephants, one oft-cited example, have at least twenty copies of it, and their cancer-free status is attributed to their TP53 advantage (scientists just discovered this in 2015, and it has since spurred new inquiries and cancer research).[16] We want to protect our TP53 not only from mutation but from conditions that will prevent its actions in the body. Which brings me back to antioxi-

---

*The molecule p53 has been dubbed "guardian of the genome." Earlier I called autophagy the guardian because it can limit DNA damage and chromosomal instability. Both deserve the nickname. And I think future research will discover other tumor-suppressing genes in addition to TP53.

dants. Can antioxidants cloak damage in the body that p53 and other molecular processes should be able to see to address? And can they likewise hinder autophagy? You bet.

Many antioxidants inhibit autophagy. By blocking autophagy, antioxidant compounds can increase the levels of aggregate-prone proteins associated with neurodegenerative disease. In fly and zebra fish models of Huntington's disease, for example, antioxidants exacerbate the disease and cancel out the benefits seen with autophagy-inducing agents. Thus, the potential advantages of some classes of antioxidants in neurodegenerative diseases may be compromised by their autophagy-blocking properties. This may also be true of other illnesses, not just neurodegenerative diseases, as I've outlined. So yes, we can get too much of a good thing (antioxidants), which is true of just about anything in life.

STRIKING A BALANCE

The studies on antioxidants will continue. Collectively, there are most likely just as many studies that show how they prevent cancer and have other health-promoting effects. This is a very complex area of medicine that future studies need to suss out. We can't forget that different antioxidants act differently and could be less harmful or even beneficial. Moreover, studies in lab dishes or in lab animals such as mice and rats may not be applicable to humans. We also cannot neglect the fact that each one of us is unique. My underlying DNA and risk of developing certain diseases is not the same as yours. Again, future researchers will figure this out and bring truly personalized medicine to market.

I think we can all agree that megadosing on anything is not good for us. It should come as no surprise that we must strike a fine balance between internal and external antioxidants. I'm going to help you do that next by giving you a program to follow. Given what we know, I think the right balance entails consuming antioxidants while you're in the feeding (anabolic) state and avoiding them when you dial up your autophagy in the catabolic (fasting) state.

My whole point of showcasing the stories in this chapter, however, is to underscore some of the nuances to life—and aging. We don't have all the answers yet, but we can learn from other things in nature, from big mammals such as the bowhead whale to little mammals such as naked mole rats and even seemingly supernatural people such as Jeanne Louise Calment. I trust that the future bodes well for us mere mortals who will continue to search for the fountain of youth. In the meantime, we can put some faith in the power of intermittent fasting, protein cycling, and ketosis. I'll also suggest you balance yourself out with exercise and stress reduction.

Let's get to it.

CHAPTER 9

FINGER PRICKS AND GROCERY LISTS

Forget juice cleanses and detox diets, teas, and elixirs. Ditch the low-fat life and infomercial gimmicks. You know the keys to living a longer, healthier life. If you haven't already begun to change a few habits based on what you've read, now is your chance. I want to make this as easy and effortless for you as possible, so in this chapter I've got a gallery of guidelines you can tailor to your own life. The goal is to implement as many of the strategies I covered in the book as possible. You will catabolize (break down) your tissues and cells eight months of the year to clean your body's house by turning autophagy up, and you will anabolize (put together or construct) your tissues and regenerate cells during the other four months by turning mTOR up, arranged whatever way suits you: two months with autophagy on and one month off, four on and two off, or even eight in a row on and four in a row off. There's no consensus on a perfect catabolic-anabolic pattern to follow, but in lieu of new studies, I think the 8-to-4 ratio is the healthiest. I will provide general principles that we would all do well to follow and then offer ideas to accelerate and maximize your results.

You've learned more about cell metabolism than most people today, including many practicing doctors, understand. Once you begin to make these changes, you will see—and feel—results quickly. If you have never tried a low-carb or keto diet, you may experience a breaking-in period during which you might feel flu-ish, drained, and generally not well. As I mentioned in chapter 5, that's perfectly normal and expected. Remember, we are reteaching your body a long-forgotten process in your metabolism. We are clearing out the clutter and stirring up some dust in the process. The body is going through a renovation of sorts that has some effects that you will feel. Focus on what's right around the corner: being more energetic, mentally clear, and vibrant. The symptoms of any chronic condition you may be living with will wane or even vanish. You will be able to sleep better, be more productive at work, and find the motivation to exercise. Not only will you gain better control of your blood sugar, levels of inflammation, weight, and chronic conditions, but you will simultaneously see changes happen in other areas of your life. You'll gain more self-confidence and navigate through stressful periods more easily.

I should reiterate that if you're currently dealing with a health condition, including pregnancy or lactation, or if you're taking medication to prevent or treat a condition, you should speak with your physician about incorporating any of the ideas and suggestions in this chapter. This is not meant to be a one-size-fits-all protocol. My hope is that you find your sweet spot in which you can reap the benefits of these strategies and adapt them as needed to lead a healthier life and live as long and well as possible.

If you're like most people, your body is addicted to carbs and swimming in too much insulin. It doesn't help that nutrition guidelines still promote the idea that we should be getting most of our calories from carbohydrates. The original Food Pyramid Guide published by the US Department of Agriculture in 1980—and its iterations since—has been destructive to our bodies and our waistlines (it's now called MyPlate). The absurdity and irony of these guidelines is that although there's such a thing as essential fats and essential amino acids, there's no such thing as essential carbohydrates, yet it's the one thing they push! Even with zero carbs coming into your body through food, you can still make glucose through the process of gluconeogenesis. The liver will convert glycerol derived from fats into glucose. Study after study has shown that people who eat a low-carb diet and do not reduce their total calories lose more weight than those who eat a low-fat diet and reduce their overall calorie consumption. That also speaks volumes.

Don't even second-guess your ability to do this; it's what we evolved to do. And don't worry about restricting your calories, cutting back on protein, and losing your love of bagels and ice cream. I realize that for many people, evicting sugar and carbs such as pastries, pancakes, and pizza can be tough. Change is hard, but monumental change has its ways of working out when you commit to the challenge and reap the rewards. On this plan, you will not feel deprived or have unbearable cravings. Take the initial plunge. But first, let's discuss some tests that will help you know whether your new lifestyle is working. This will also give you a baseline at the start.

FINGER PRICKS

What's the result of a lifetime of keeping the gas pedal for mTOR floored while keeping the brake for autophagy pulled? If you live in the first world, the risk of your becoming obese or developing diabetes, heart disease, cancer, and/or Alzheimer's disease (and many people do develop more than one of these at a time, called comorbidity) is mind-boggling, whereas, as we've seen, those who follow a more "primitive" diet in health oases such as Okinawa, Loma Linda, and Mount Athos are at a far lower level of risk of developing these diseases of civilization. Turning up the Switch and restoring autophagy to the level of our Paleolithic ancestors' is how we stack the deck in our favor. It's how we can fine-tune the body's system and perhaps reverse the course of a disease or entirely prevent one from taking root.

When starting a new health regimen, I'm a big fan of self-quantification, keeping track of your health parameters including weight, BMI, muscle mass, vascular adipose tissue, bone density, and various blood chemistry markers. Self-quantification will help you monitor your risk factors (high blood glucose, hypertension, high triglycerides or cholesterol, and so on). It will also give you feedback on how following the practices I outline, such as eating more whole plants and less animal meat and dairy products (but not necessarily animal fat) and fasting, is working to improve those health markers and lower your disease risks. The test results will give you a baseline and can further motivate you to change your behavior and take control of your well-being.

Medicine now has the ability to profile you to determine your risk of developing certain diseases—from obesity and diabetes to Alzheimer's and cancer. The laboratory studies listed in this chapter are available today, are economical, and are covered by most insurance plans. Many can even be performed in a pharmacy that includes a clinic and can be done by a registered nurse. I do, however, recommend that if you are currently managing any condition, schedule a visit with your physician so you can have all of your diagnostic tests evaluated by him or her. You will want to have a conversation about the lifestyle changes you plan to make within the context of any medical condition, including pregnancy, that you are treating. This is especially true if you currently take medications. You may also want to go ahead and have a full physical, making sure that you get all of these tests performed in addition to any others that your doctor recommends. If you have a family history of a certain illness, such as dementia or diabetes, you'll want to speak with your doctor about that and ask if there are additional tests you can take or ways of further preventing such a diagnosis for you.

Now that DNA sequencing has gone mass market and is widely available through various biotechnology companies, I encourage you to obtain your personal genomics and risk profile. You can buy DNA test kits at pharmacies or through an online search; all you do is spit into a tube and mail the package to the biotechnology company. Though some of the data can be more entertaining than informative, such as telling you what type of earwax you have or your genetic ancestry, some of the data can reveal genetic variants that make you more susceptible for certain conditions. But remember that your DNA sequence is just one part of the puzzle. DNA says more about your risk than your fate. Your DNA sequence foretells probabilities, for the most part, not necessarily your destiny. And how our DNA is expressed has more to do with your lifestyle choices than the genetic cards you were dealt at birth. Put simply, you can change your body's destiny by the way you eat, sleep, move, and breathe. Now let's get to those tests, all of which should be repeated during regular annual checkups.

+ **Fasting blood glucose:** I recommend buying an inexpensive glucose meter (and aim for strips that cost less than a dollar a day). These can be purchased online or at your local pharmacy. Use it first thing upon waking every day, and mark your result on a calendar. I put this on my online calendar along with a daily description of what and how much I eat throughout the day so that I can go back and decipher what's improving or throwing off my desired morning level. Your morning result is typically affected by what you ate the day before. A commonly used diagnostic tool to check for prediabetes and diabetes, a blood glucose monitor measures the amount of sugar (glucose) in your blood after you have not eaten for at least eight hours. A fasting level between 70 and 100 milligrams per deciliter (mg/dL) is considered normal; above this, your body is showing signs of insulin resistance and diabetes and an increased risk of developing brain disease. Ideally, you want to have a fasting blood glucose of less than 95 mg/dL. I try to keep my personal fasting (morning) blood glucose level around 75 to 85 mg/dL. Otherwise, you'll be keeping your autophagy switch off. You can also check your level one hour after consuming a meal or snack. If it's over 120 mg/dL, either you consumed too much or you need fewer high-glycemic carbs in your next meal.

✦ **Hemoglobin A1c:** As I explained earlier, this test reveals an "average" blood sugar level over a ninety-day period, and as such, it provides a far better indication of overall blood sugar control. It's a commonly used test in doctor's offices during routine exams. A good A1c value is between 4.8 and 5.4 percent. A value between 5.7 and 6.4 percent indicates prediabetes, and 6.5 percent or above indicates full-blown diabetes. It can take time to see this number improve, which is why it's typically measured only once every three to four months (or annually at routine physicals). The autophagy switch cannot be dialed up if your A1c level is chronically high.

✦ **Homocysteine:** A higher level of this amino acid, which is produced by the body, is associated with many conditions, from atherosclerosis (narrowing and hardening of the arteries), heart disease, and stroke to renal disease, depression, and dementia. People who consume a lot of meat and dairy products tend to score high because those foods contain methionine, an amino acid that is converted to homocysteine in the body. Your level should be 10 millimole per liter (μmol/L) or less. Note that a high level of homocysteine has also been shown to triple the rate of telomere shortening. Telomeres are the "caps" on the ends of your chromosomes that protect your genes; their length is a biological indication of how fast you are aging. You will automatically lower your homocysteine levels once you cut back on your consumption of meat and dairy products. Exercise and certain B vitamins, notably folate (B_9), B_{12}, B_6, and B_2, can also help lower your level. The body relies on these vitamins to metabolize homocysteine, which is why people with a high homocysteine level also tend to be low in B vitamins.

✦ **C-reactive protein (CRP):** This is a marker of inflammation. You want to see 0.00 to 3.0 milligrams per liter (mg/L). Your CRP level may take several months to improve, but you may well see positive changes even after one month on my plan.

✦ **Lipid profile (or lipid panel):** This measures the amount of cholesterol (LDL and HDL as well as total cholesterol) and triglycerides in the blood. Triglycerides are a type of fat in the blood, and high levels often indicate a problem with the liver or pancreas. High levels tend to show up with other problems such as diabetes, obesity, high blood pressure, and an unhealthy balance of HDL/LDL cholesterol. Too much refined sugar and alcohol will raise your triglyceride levels. According to the Cleveland Clinic, here are your target numbers:[*]

- ❖ **Total cholesterol:** 100–199 mg/dL (for those over age 21)

- ❖ **High-density lipoprotein (HDL):** Greater than 40 mg/dL

- ❖ **Low-density lipoprotein (LDL):** Less than 70 mg/dL for those with heart or blood ves-

---

[*]These target values are different for children and teens. Newer methods of evaluating cholesterol levels and related health risks are beginning to emerge. One, for example, is called the Martin-Hopkins equation and is supposed to help doctors more precisely calculate an LDL value without the patient needing to fast before the blood is drawn. But most health centers still use the reference points listed above.

sel disease and for other people at very high risk of heart disease (those with metabolic syndrome). Less than 100 mg/dL for high-risk patients (e.g., some patients who have multiple heart disease risk factors). Less than 130 mg/dL for individuals who are at low risk for coronary artery disease.

❖ **Triglycerides:** Less than 150 mg/dL.

✦ **Omega-6-to-omega-3 ratio:** As previously noted, you can check your level of omega-3s through a simple blood test you can do at home with a kit you purchase online. This is not a typical test that your doctor will order unless you ask. You'll want an omega-3 index in the range of 8 to 12 percent. In terms of the ratio of omega-6 to omega-3, you'll want it to be in the range of 2 to 1 to 1 to 1.

✦ **DEXA scan:** This low-dose X-ray procedure, which takes about ten minutes, is becoming increasingly popular around the United States. DEXA stands for **d**ual-**e**nergy **X**-ray **a**bsorptiometry, which is a fancy term for the technology used to scan the body noninvasively. Look for companies that offer whole-body imaging and not just bone density scans. Many companies provide 3-D scans that will give you your BMI, percentage of body fat, muscle mass, and bone density region by region. You can use these scans to get short-term feedback on how your diet is doing, whether you're gaining or losing muscle, and whether you need to boost your calcium and vitamin K_2 supplementation and/or engage in weight-bearing exercises to build up your bone density. These scans can be done through your doctor, or, depending on where you live, you can find medical imaging centers that provide them. You do not need a prescription, and they cost as little as $45.

After three months in the program, aim to repeat these tests to note any improvements. Then request them during your annual visit with your doctor.

TEN KEYS TO THE SWITCH LIFESTYLE

Now's a good time to recap what you've learned so far. Here are the ten key facts to remember:

1. Animals, yeast, protozoa, and plants all experience feast (anabolic) and famine (catabolic) states, and their mTOR switch turns on and off as ours does, switching from growth (anabolic) to recycling (catabolic).

2. From the time our earliest ancestors began hunting and gathering on the African savanna until the start of the Agricultural Revolution roughly 12 thousand

years ago, about 4 million years passed. Thus, humans have been consuming grains and dairy products for less than one-fourth of 1 percent of our time on Earth; put another way, we've spent about four hundred times longer as hunter-gatherers than we have as farmers or ranchers.

3. Your caveman ancestors most likely consumed low-glycemic grasses, seeds, nuts, and tubers, as much fat as they could get, and meat, when available. They consumed honey and grains seasonally, but neither was a substantial contributor to their daily calories.

4. The diseases of civilization (diabetes, cancer, cardiovascular diseases, and Alzheimer's disease) started occurring in a far greater percentage of the population whenever societies switched from hunter-gatherer to grain-based diets, especially after the advent of refined, mass-produced sugars and flours.

5. Numerous groups around the world, including the Okinawans, Loma Linda vegans, and Mount Athos monks, eschew the Western diet, eat more whole plants and less meat and dairy products, and enjoy longer lives with far lower levels of diabetes, cancer, cardiovascular disease, and Alzheimer's disease than do those following a typical Western diet, which

is high in refined grains, sugars, and farmed meat products.

6. Consuming less animal protein and dairy products lowers IGF-1 levels (as experienced by all three groups listed earlier, similar to Laron syndrome dwarfs, who have loss-of-function IGF-1 receptor genes), which turns down mTOR. This is how one enters a catabolic state, in which autophagy turns up and your body cleans out misfolded proteins and dysfunctional organelles.

7. Consuming fewer high-glycemic carbs (i.e., sugars, flours, easily digested starches, and many fruits) will lower your blood glucose level, protecting you from advanced glycation end products (AGEs) and turning down mTOR.

8. Consuming a low enough level of carbohydrates (less than 20 grams a day), so that you continually produce ketones and are thus in a ketogenic state, not only turns down mTOR but can aid to improve your brain function, enable you to fast more easily, and help you burn fat to improve your health and lose weight faster.

9. Try to choose foods that are anti-inflammatory and avoid those that are pro-inflammatory (e.g., avoid

foods high in omega-6 fatty acids and increase your intake of omega-3 fatty acids).

10. The key to long-term good health is cycling your diet so that you're in a catabolic state about eight months out of the year and an anabolic state the other four months. Following this pattern (however you want to break it down—eight straight months or two out of every three months) will most accurately mimic your ancestral dietary cycles and provide sufficient "house-cleaning" to greatly reduce your risk of developing diseases of civilization while providing your body with periods of renewed growth of stem cells and a stronger immune system while replenishing muscle and some fat.

GO AHEAD AND TURN THE SWITCH

Here is a list of general guidelines for your eight-months-per-year autophagy-inducing catabolic state. Later, I'll suggest that you also choose a lifestyle group (Okinawans, Loma Linda vegans, or Mount Athos monks) to mimic, which will help you organize your dietary habits around a theme (low calorie, low protein, or frequent fasts). Another option for your eight-month catabolic state, which I'll discuss later, will be to follow a ketogenic diet, which I personally think is more powerful for dieting and getting down to your ideal BMI.

✦ **Evict the refined carbs.** Cereal, chips, crackers, cookies, pasta, pastries, muffins, cakes, doughnuts, sugary snacks, candy, energy bars, ice cream, ketchup, processed cheese spreads, juices, sports drinks, soft drinks/soda, fried foods, and all packaged foods, especially those labeled "fat free" or "low fat." Ditch all "natural" sugars, too, such as honey, molasses, brown sugar, agave, maple syrup, and table sugar. Nix all artificial sweeteners and sugar substitutes as well, and products made with them (you can get a touch of sweetness from stevia and monk fruit).

✦ **Eat more whole-food plants.** Focus on low-glycemic vegetables and legumes (when in doubt, check online at any of the many databases; Harvard Health, for example, maintains an updated list). Note that flash-frozen and canned produce is fine as long as there are no added sugars, preservatives, or other ingredients.

❖ **Unlimited:** Mushrooms, cauliflower, arugula, green beans, peas, lentils, chickpeas, yams (not white potatoes), cabbage, lettuce, endive, brussels sprouts, kale, chard, onions, collards, bok choy, artichokes, celery, radishes, asparagus, garlic, leeks, fennel, shallots, scallions, ginger, jicama, parsley, water chestnuts.

❖ **Smaller portions/less frequently (due to their high oxalate* content):** Spinach, broccoli, white potatoes/sweet potatoes, eggplant.

✦ **Eat a lot less animal protein, including eggs and dairy products (but excluding omega-3-rich fish).** Try to limit your weekly meat intake to 8 ounces or less and stop consuming milk, except for occasional "feast" goat's or sheep's milk or cheese (not more than once a week; more on this below). Buy pastured eggs and consume them in moderation (no more than two per week).

✦ **Eat a lot fewer foods (bread and pasta) containing whole grains, such as wheat, barley, rye, etc., and stay away from refined flour entirely.** Try to limit the bread and pasta to once a week or less. An exception is low-glycemic lupin, which is high in protein and fiber and low in net carbs (i.e., total carbs minus fiber). You may have never heard of it until now, but it's gaining popularity and is widely

---

*Oxalate crystals are present in most plant foods to varying degrees. The large microcrystals have the potential to inflict mechanical injury, whereas the ionic, soluble, and nanocrystal forms of oxalate are readily absorbed and wreak havoc throughout the body. Oxalates are associated with pain and both functional and chronic disorders. For more information, see Sally K. Norton, "Lost Seasonality and Overconsumption of Plants: Risking Oxalate Toxicity," *Journal of Evolution and Health* 2, no. 3 (May 2018): article 4, https://jevohealth.com/journal/vol2/iss3/4/ or https://sallyknorton.com/downloads/lost -seasonality-risking-oxalate-toxicity/.

available online or in most grocery stores. It's actually a legume and a substitute for flour. You can buy lupin "flour" and bake cookies and pancakes with it instead of regular flour. You can also buy lupin flakes and toss them in salads or coat fish with them before panfrying. If you can cut other cereal grains out of your diet completely, you'll be better off.

+ **Eat more macadamia nuts** (up to 4 ounces a day, or about 48 nuts), and try to consume all other nuts, such as almonds, cashews, peanuts, pine nuts, and most seeds, in moderation. It's hard to overeat nuts, and I'd rather you be eating them over processed foods. But when choosing nuts, opt for macadamias first.

+ **Eat oils that are high in monounsaturated fats** (e.g., avocado, macadamia nut, and extra-virgin olive oil), including as a dressing on salads.

+ **Skip breakfast as frequently as possible to give yourself more overnight fasting time.** Start with a twelve-hour overnight fast (that is, no calories between 6:00 p.m. and 6:00 a.m.), and, by skipping breakfast, work yourself up to an eighteen-hour fast at least three days a week (that is, no calories between 6:00 p.m. and noon).

✦ **Activate autophagy through protein cycling.**
Choose three nonconsecutive low-protein days
(e.g., Monday, Wednesday, Friday), fast overnight
and into the morning (for a total of eighteen hours,
ideally), and then limit your protein intake for the
remainder of the day to no more than 25 grams
(the equivalent of 8 medium shrimp, 4.4 ounces
of salmon, or 3 ounces of roast turkey or chicken
breast). For the remaining four days of the week,
you can have a normal protein intake (roughly
0.37 grams per each pound of body weight; so a
150-pound individual can consume 55 grams of
protein).

✦ **Learn to do one-, then two-, then three-to-five-
day fasts from once a month to once a quarter**
(depending on your health and weight goals).
One strategy that many people swear by is to go
into ketosis for one month, followed by a five-
day fast. For those who struggle with weight and
metabolic conditions, this could be a solution to
both goals.

✦ **Follow nature's cues and become seasonal.** Start
eating more carbs, fruits, and meat in the late sum-
mer/early fall during the months when you should
be outside absorbing more sunlight (vitamin D).
Allow yourself to put on a little more weight going

into the winter, and then fast more frequently during the winter and/or go keto during those months (more on keto on the following page).

LIFESTYLES

Choose any one of the following styles of eating *while still abiding by the general guidelines just given*:

- ✦ **Eat like the Okinawans.** Lower your calorie intake by picking an ideal body weight and consuming just enough calories to maintain that (aim to consume your basal metabolic rate's worth of calories while you're trying to reach your ideal weight). Lots of online websites will calculate this for you. If you don't know how many calories you consume in a day, track them by logging everything you eat and using an online calculator to add them up. Eat far less animal protein each week, and focus on plant-based meals. Cut out processed meats (no bacon or hot dogs). Whenever possible, go for fatty fish such as salmon, halibut, sardines, or black cod instead of omega-6-packed poultry and livestock.

- ✦ **Eat like monks.** Restrict your calories and go low-glycemic vegan half the time (180 days a year, which can be every other week or, ideally, every other month). The other half of the time, you can have animal protein (especially fish) and more carbs than on your restricted-calorie days.

+ **Eat like Loma Linda vegans.** Restrict all animal protein, but supplement with B vitamins and extra veggie proteins such as textured vegetable protein (TVP). TVP is a substitute for meat and can be found in the bulk foods section of many natural foods stores and the baking aisles of grocery stores. It has a similar texture to ground meat when cooked and can be incorporated into soups, stews, and vegetarian tacos, casseroles, and veggie burgers. I throw it into a lot of dishes.

+ **Go keto.** Switch your body to burning primarily fats two out of every three months or every other month. Dropping carbs will help turn up autophagy and also make it much easier to do fasts, since your body will continue using fat (but your own rather than the fats you eat), preventing you from experiencing hunger the way you would when kicking carbs. The combination of being in keto and dialing up autophagy is a win-win for your whole metabolism.

SAMPLE CALENDAR YEAR

JANUARY: Autophagy month

FEBRUARY: Autophagy month (option: with keto)

MARCH: Anabolic (dial-down) month

APRIL: Autophagy month

MAY: Autophagy month (option: with keto)

JUNE: Anabolic (dial-down) month

JULY: Autophagy month

AUGUST: Autophagy month (option: with keto)

SEPTEMBER: Anabolic (dial-down) month with more flexibility for feast days

OCTOBER: Autophagy month

NOVEMBER: Autophagy month (option: with keto)

DECEMBER: Anabolic (dial-down) month

Note: You get to choose how to map out your year. Aim for eight months with autophagy dialed up and four months with it dialed down to rebuild cells and tissues. Go keto during some of the autophagy months. Use a month during the fall to give yourself some more feast days in preparation for winter.

GROCERY LIST

Note: Try to buy organic foods whenever possible. Remember, the goal is to make every meal mostly plant based. You will no longer design meals around protein and carbs with a "side salad." On the contrary, plants will become your centerpiece and you can occasionally add animal proteins—up to 8 ounces a week. The animal proteins will essentially become your "side" dish for two meals a week during the months you're in autophagy. (Let's give you a feast day once a month, however, during which you can eat whatever you want. Even during the months in autophagy, one day off won't kill the program.)

- Low-glycemic produce (e.g., lettuce, mushrooms, cauliflower, cucumbers, green beans, brussels sprouts, chard, onions, collards, leeks, scallions, artichokes, radishes, asparagus, zucchini, acorn squash, yellow squash, garlic, ginger, tomatoes, avocados, blueberries, raspberries, blackberries, kale, yams, lemons)

- Herbs and spices (e.g., oregano, parsley, thyme, mint, basil, turmeric, cinnamon)

- Macadamia nuts and macadamia nut butter

- DHA-enhanced pastured eggs

- Cold-water fatty wild fish (e.g., salmon, halibut, sardines, mackerel, anchovies)

- Canned tuna (pole-caught)

- Shrimp

- Hempseed

- Flaxseed

- Chia seeds

- Lupin flakes or flour

- Extra-virgin olive oil

- Coconut or MCT oil

- Avocado oil and mayo

- Dijon mustard

- Tapenade (no added sugar)

- Salsa (no added sugar)

- Plain (unsweetened) sheep's milk full-fat yogurt

- Hummus

- Lentils

- Chickpeas

- Black beans

- Sea salt or Himalayan pink salt

- Balsamic vinegar

- Dark chocolate (at least 70 percent cacao)

- Stevia or monk fruit for sweetness

- Coffee, tea

HOW TO GO KETO

The most important strategy in going keto is to drastically reduce your carb consumption. For most people, this means keeping net carbs, defined as digestible carbs (total carbs minus fiber), under 50 grams per day and ideally below 20 grams. You can do the math yourself by using the listed ingredients on any packaged food; for whole foods you buy without a label, just look them up online. The numbers are everywhere now. The fewer the carbs, the better. You will replace carb calories with healthy fats and proteins, though the fats will take up the majority of your diet (again, no processed meats such bacon or sausage—lots of keto plans allow these, but they are not healthy sources of nutrition). Remember, protein can be converted to blood sugar in the body, and too much protein is not good for you. The carbs that you do consume should come from aboveground vegetables such as lettuce, cucumbers, mushrooms, cauliflower, asparagus, and cabbage (no potatoes, carrots, yams, or sweet potatoes). Also avoid carb-heavy legumes such as peas, lentils, and beans. Fruits are difficult to consume and still stay in keto due to their sugar content (a single piece of sweet fruit can deliver 20 or more grams of carbs). You can eat berries occasionally but no bananas, peaches, or pineapple.

I use MyFitnessPal, but there are lots of online resources and phone apps to help you count carbs and keep track of your protein and fat consumption at the start so you can learn how to stay within the parameters for a healthy ketogenic diet. The app is great for scanning bar codes and so you know exactly what the quantities of nutrients in a food are and to keep track of your calories (you won't be buying much packaged food anymore, but if you buy frozen or canned veggies, for example, those codes come in handy). MyFitnessPal also maintains a website so you can know what's in your meals, including restaurant meals. While on the keto diet, supplement with B vitamins and fish oil.

SHEEP OVER COWS

Cow's milk dominates many people's diets. Dairy products are pervasive in our culture—from breakfast to dinner and in-between snacks. We add them to coffee and consume them in the form of ice cream, yogurt, and cheese. A much better alternative is sheep's milk. Sheep's milk is more acceptable to the human digestive system than cow's milk. It's even better digested than goat's milk. And a bonus: sheep's milk does not have a strong smell or taste, as is often the case with goat's milk. As part of the Switch dietary protocol, you can consume sheep's milk and cheese made from sheep's milk. (Sheep's milk is actually ideal for cheese production because it contains double the amount of solids of cow's or goat's milk.) For autophagy purposes, it has far less leucine than cow's milk but is still inappropriate to consume during your eight months' catabolic phase. You should consume sheep's milk only when you're in your anabolic phase, but try to avoid cow's and goat's milk except for special occasions, which occur only a few times a year.

COOK WITH HEALTHY OILS

I like to cook with coconut, avocado, and extra-virgin olive oils. I'll also use a high-quality canola oil cooking spray when using high heat. And I like to use olive oil liberally for its healthy omega-3 fat content. It's my go-to for cooking and for drizzling over raw or prepared food.

DRINK UP

Try to stick with purified water, drinking half of your body weight in ounces daily. If you weigh 150 pounds, that means drinking at least 75 ounces of water per day. I do recommend coffee in the morning if you're a coffee drinker, but please no added sugar or milk. You can also opt for tea. On feast days, which are like special occasions for holidays and celebrations (about once a month), you can have a glass of wine with dinner. Avoid alcohol if you're in keto.

SNACKING

You probably won't find yourself hungry between meals, but if you do, go for a handful of macadamia nuts or chopped raw low-glycemic vegetables such as celery and radishes dipped in tapenade, fresh salsa, hummus, or guacamole. Try half an avocado with olive oil drizzled on top, salt, and pepper. Or cook an artichoke and dip the leaves into avocado mayo.

EATING OUT

I recommend that you avoid eating out during the first few weeks of changing your dietary life. Too many temptations are out there, and you know it. Eventually, however, you will need to figure out how to maintain this lifestyle wherever you are. I realize that it's virtually impossible to plan and prepare every single meal and snack you eat, and you are probably regularly faced with tempta-tion (e.g., buffets, commissaries, lunch meetings, birthday parties, Thanksgiving). See if you can return to your favorite restaurants and order from the menu while still following this protocol. And once you've gotten used to this way of eating, you can return to your old recipes and modify them to fit my guidelines. It's not that hard to make any menu or recipe work for you as long as you're savvy about your choices. When in doubt, I often go for an arugula salad with avocado, drizzled with oil and vinegar. If I'm doing keto, I can add some seafood (not battered) to the salad.

IN SUM

I created this visual to help you see the gist of the entire protocol. I don't expect you to follow it to a T, but do the best you can. Note that macadamia nuts are a source of both healthy fat and protein, which is why I love them so much.

The Switch Food Plan

(in order of calories consumed)

Healthy Fats: 7 days a week		
(65–75% of calories, macadamia nut, avocado, MCT, olive, or canola)		
Low-Glycemic Vegetables: 7 days a week		
(10–25% of calories, brussel sprouts, cauliflower, spinach, broccoli, kale, yellow squash, onions)		
Vegetable Proteins (except soy): 7 days a week		
(not to exceed 10% of calories, hemp protein, pea protein, macadamia nuts)		
Vegan Only: 3–7 days a week (above foods)	**Fatty Fish: 0–3 days a week** (salmon, sardines, shrimp)	**Dairy and Meat: 0–1 day a week** (preferably grass-fed, and in moderation)
Sweets, Grains, Legumes, Starches, Nuts		
(only during the fall [August–Sept] or on feast days, less than 25% of calories)		
Alcohol: 1–2 Drinks/Day on Feast Days Only		
(preferably red wine, but any alcohol is allowed; no fruit or added sugar if doing keto)		
Fasting		
(3 consecutive days, quarterly)		

SUPPLEMENTS TO CONSIDER

If you currently take any prescription medication, it's important that you consult with your physician before starting any supplement program. Talk about the risks versus benefits and factor the conditions you are currently treating into your decisions about which supplements to take. Don't forget to include over-the-counter medications and supplements that you take as well.

Below is my list of the top four drugs and supplements you might want to add to your regimen. They are chosen because they relate directly to autophagy.

+ **Aspirin:** This long-established analgesic has potent anti-inflammatory effects in the body. The "wonder drug" also induces autophagy because its active metabolite—salicylate—inhibits mTOR, which is why it is called a mimic to calorie restriction. The decision to take a low-dose "baby" aspirin (81 mg) daily is one to make with your doctor given your health history, age, and personal risks. Aspirin can promote spontaneous bleeding and prevent certain people from clotting properly. It is not recommended for everyone.

+ **Vitamin D:** It's a misnomer to call vitamin D a vitamin because it's actually a fat-soluble steroid hormone and we have a built-in technology for producing it. The body naturally manufactures vitamin D from cholesterol in the skin upon exposure to UV rays from the sun. Although most people associate it with bone health and calcium levels—hence its addition to fortified foods and beverages—it has far-reaching effects on the body and stimulates autophagy. Autophagy is in fact a basis of the health-promoting effects of vitamin D—the body *requires* vitamin D to fulfill its autophagy duties (perhaps this is why there are receptors for vitamin D throughout the body). Vitamin D deficiency is associated with an increased risk of developing a multitude of health challenges, from weak, soft bones and, at the extreme end, osteoporosis and rickets to diabetes, depression, dementia, and cardiovascular disease. A lot of us are deficient in this vitamin because we shun the sun or live in northern latitudes where adequate sun exposure is difficult throughout much of the year. Testing for vitamin D levels is no longer recommended because the meaning of the results has been called into question. It's safe to assume that you can boost your levels, and it doesn't hurt to supplement with 2,000 IU daily. You can't overdose at that level, even if you do get plenty of sunscreen-free sunshine.

✦ **Fish oil (DHA and EPA):** These omega-3 stars often come together. If you're vegan, you can buy them derived from marine algae (the reason fish oil contains so much omega-3 is that the fishes' main source of food is algae).

✦ **Glucosamine:** This supplement, commonly used to help repair joint problems such as osteoarthritis, is a strong autophagy inducer independent of the mTOR pathway (meaning it works separately from other mTOR-inhibiting practices and can be combined during your catabolic phase to increase autophagy activation).

Here's a list of some other autophagy-inducing nutraceuticals that you might consider taking *only during your catabolic phase*. Follow the recommended dosages on the packages.

✦ *Astragalus membranaceus* (Huang Qi)

✦ **Ashwagandha**, a water extract of ashwagandha leaves

✦ **Caffeine**, taken as additional coffee, but not enough to interfere with your sleep

✦ **Carnosic acid and carnosol** (polyphenols from rosemary)

✦ **Turmeric or curcumin**

+ **Epigallocatechin gallate (EGCG)**, a major component of green tea

+ **Fisetin**, a naturally occurring flavonoid found in several fruits and vegetables

+ **Ginger root**, sliced or ground (not candied)

+ **Indole-3-carbinol**, an extract from cruciferous vegetables such as broccoli, cabbage, cauliflower, brussels sprouts, collard greens, and kale

+ **Melatonin**, a hormone produced naturally by the body but available over the counter as a supplement

+ **Nicotinic acid (aka niacin)**, vitamin B_3

+ **Pterostilbene**, a plant stilbenoid related to, but more powerful than, resveratrol

+ **Pycnogenol (aka French maritime pine bark extract)**, a standardized extract from the bark of a tree

+ **Quercetin**, a plant flavonol from the flavonoid group of polyphenols, found in many fruits, vegetables, leaves, grains, red onions, and kale

+ **Resveratrol**, a stilbenoid, a type of natural phenol produced by various plants in response to injury or when the plant is under attack by pathogens such as bacteria or fungi

Autophagy-inducing pharmaceuticals include:

- **Metformin:** A drug that interferes with the mitochondria's electron transport chain to reduce the amount of cellular energy (ATP) produced, which signals AMPK (see chapter 3) to put the brakes on cell division and protein production by inhibiting mTOR. Take this only under the supervision of a doctor and only while in your catabolic phase.

- **Rapamycin:** This drug is derived from the bacteria we discussed in the first part of this book, which led to the discovery of mTOR. It is prescribed to suppress the immune system after certain types of transplants; this will strongly inhibit mTOR and should be taken only under the supervision of a doctor, and only while in your catabolic phase.

POWER UP AUTOPHAGY WITH EXERCISE

We all know that exercise is good for us, even if many of us don't engage in it enough. But could it be that the main reason it's so beneficial is that it induces autophagy? Exercise is a known stimulator of autophagy in both muscle tissues and the brain. In one particularly illuminating 2012 study done at the University of

Texas Southwestern Medical Center, researchers engineered mice to have glowing green autophagosomes, the structures that form around the pieces of cells that the body has decided to recycle.[1] The rate at which the mice healthily demolished their own cells increased sharply after they ran for thirty minutes on a treadmill. Thirty minutes of running increased autophagy by 40 to 50 percent. And the rate continued increasing until they'd been running for eighty minutes, at which point autophagy was increased to 100 percent (don't panic: you don't have to exercise for eighty minutes a day). This study, published in the prestigious journal *Nature*, was led by Dr. Beth Levine, who had already made a name for herself in autophagy research. In 1999, she found the first mammalian autophagy gene and discovered the link between a defect in that gene and breast cancer.[2] She also helped in using the research worm *C. elegans* to show that autophagy plays a role in life span extension.[3]

Until her *Nature* paper, the best known way to induce autophagy in mice was to stress them with starvation for forty-eight hours. Not only is exercise another form of stress on the body that stimulates autophagy, but it's even faster than starvation. What's really interesting about her study is that she and her colleagues fed the mice a high-fat diet to create diabetes associated with obesity and then gave the mice eight weeks of daily training running on the treadmill. (Note to clarify: A high-fat diet for mice is never ketogenic and has enough carbs to keep the body burning glucose only and storing all of the additional fat the mice eat.) The result? Compared to mutant mice that could not induce higher levels of autophagy with exercise, the normal mice reversed their diabetes. Her results were so compelling that she was inspired to buy a treadmill.

Studies in humans are still under way, and we don't know yet the ideal level of exercise or type to determine what triggers autophagy. But I think it's safe to say that maintaining a regular exercise program is essential to good health. And I know I'm not the first person to tell you that. Exercise has a synergistic effect on the body. It helps set the stage for powering up autophagy by balancing your blood sugar level, lowering your inflammation level, and burning energy so your body is forced to turn to fat for fuel. Unlike so many other claims out there in health circles, exercise is not quack medicine.

Aim to engage in aerobic physical activity if you're not already doing so for a minimum of twenty minutes a day. Get your heart rate up to at least 50 percent of your resting baseline. Don't be afraid to sweat. Force your lungs and heart to work harder. If you've been leading a primarily sedentary lifestyle, simply go for a twenty-minute walk each day and add more minutes as you get comfortable with your routine. You can add intensity to your walk by increasing your speed and finding inclines. Or carry a five-pound free weight in each hand and perform some biceps curls as you walk.

If you already maintain a fitness regimen, increase your workouts to a minimum of thirty minutes a day at least five days a week. If you're not self-motivated to exercise, enlist a friend to work out with you or try a group fitness class. You don't have to join a traditional gym. These days, opportunities to exercise are everywhere, and they needn't be costly. You can even stream videos and exercise in the comfort of your own home.

A comprehensive workout ideally should include a balanced mix of cardiovascular exercises, strength training, and stretching.

But if you're starting from scratch, establish a cardio base first and add strength training and stretching over time. Once you've gotten a regular workout down, you can schedule your daily routines around different types of exercise. Plan your exercise in advance as you would other commitments in your life. If you know you're entering a busy week and finding time to devote to formal exercise will be difficult, think about the ways you can get in more minutes of physical activity throughout the day. All the research indicates that you can get similar health benefits from doing three ten-minute bursts of exercise as you would from doing a single thirty-minute workout. Also think of ways to combine physical movement with other tasks: conducting a meeting while walking outside, for instance, or watching television while stretching. If possible, limit the time you spend sitting down. That's the most important takeaway from the latest research on exercise. "Sitting disease" is no joke.

SLEEP AND STRESS REDUCTION

I'm not going to say much about sleep because the topic is deserving of its own book. But sleep is finally gaining the spotlight in medicine thanks to the explosion of research into its profound effects on our bodies—physically, mentally, and emotionally. We need sleep to survive, period. We even need it to support autophagy. Sleep deprivation damages our metabolism and in turn our ability to enhance autophagy. Studies show that poor sleep, especially fragmented sleep during which we miss out on restful sleep, prevents our autophagy switch from going on.[4] In fact, autophagy can occur during sleep. But if we're not routinely getting a good night's slumber, our circadian rhythm will be off. That's our body's sense of time—day and night—that regulates important biological functions and hormones. Here's the important part: not only does our circadian rhythm help control the sleep cycle, it is also linked to autophagy. Our biological clock affects the autophagy rhythm. Hence, getting a proper amount of sleep will help with autophagy, ensuring that autophagy is dialed up when it should be. In 2016, scientists found that in mice, sleep interruption negatively affected autophagy.

Fully one-third of American adults get less than the recommended seven hours of sleep a night. You may not even be aware that you have poor sleep quality.[5] If you find that despite getting enough sleep, you're still tired during the day, especially if you are male, are overweight, have high blood pressure, or have been told you snore, talk to your doctor about your sleep before turning to sleep aids. Your doctor can rule out conditions that are affecting your sleep. Sleep apnea, for example, is a common but treatable ailment characterized by nighttime pauses in breathing that disrupt your sleep cycle.

To ensure that you're doing all that you can to maximize high-quality, restful sleep, below are some tips:

> ✦ **Stick to the clock.** Experts in sleep medicine like to call this "sleep hygiene"—the ways in which we ensure refreshing sleep night after night. One of the biggest rules to follow is to go to bed and get up at the same time seven days a week, 365 days a year. Keep your bedtime routine consistent.

+ **Send sleepytime signals.** Wind down at least an hour beforehand and engage in a relaxing activity. Avoid electronics and screens that emit stimulating blue light (or use glasses that help block out this light). Take a warm bath, drink some herbal tea, pick up a book.

+ **Make it a clean sanctuary.** Try to keep your bedroom a quiet, peaceful place free of arousing hardware (TVs, computers, phones, etc.), as well as clutter. Invest in a comfortable bed and plush sheets. Maintain dim lighting.

Stress in general can be incredibly toxic to our bodies. In addition to enjoying restful sleep, which will help reduce overall stress and help you better tackle difficulties in life, find ways to control your stress. This could be any number of things, from planning quality time with friends to taking up restorative yoga or starting a gratitude journal. There is a multitude of stress-reducing activities; you just have to find what works for you and do more of it.

Every day you make thousands of decisions, many of them subconscious and in line with well-ingrained habits. Be patient with yourself as you transition to this new way of life. The whole point of this book has been to inspire you to make better decisions that will ultimately enable you to live long and vibrantly. I see the value that being healthy brings to people every day in my work and collaboration with people around the world. I also see what sudden illness and chronic diseases can do. If you don't have your health, nothing else really matters. But when you do, and you feel good about yourself and your future, anything is possible.

A HEALTHY LOVE OF LIFE

Tips from Supercentenarians:
If you keep your mind busy and keep your body
busy, you're going to be around a long time.
Morning walks and chocolate.
Raw eggs and no husband.
Reading and reciting Shakespeare.
Completing the London Times *crossword puzzle every afternoon.*
Daily calisthenics and cigars.
Two pounds of chocolate a week.
I drink a shot of whiskey every day.
Friends, drinking lots of good water, staying
positive, and lots of singing.

The above snippets came from the people I met while traveling the world collecting blood samples from supercentenarians. Clearly, many of them broke the rules of what we think makes for a good, long life. But they did have one thing in common that we all would do well to heed: they lived life to the fullest and didn't do anything too extreme. They definitely had some genetic advantages (and we've documented a few already), but they nonetheless give us new clues to aging well no matter how long we have on this planet. You can have Cadillac genes, but if you don't maintain yourself and change your metaphorical oil, you will not last as long (or look or feel as good) as the person with a well-maintained Chevy.

I don't have an aversion to death. I like to say I have a healthy love of life. And I hold a genuine deep conviction that longer lives would make humans more humane—something the world needs now more than ever before. At my Betterhumans nonprofit research organization, we strive to find the secrets of staying as healthy as possible for as long as one wants—even indefinitely. Dr. Thomas Perls is a geriatrician at Boston University who also studies superagers; he is the founder and director of the New England Centenarian Study. I think he stated the reality perfectly in a 1999 paper in *The Lancet*: "It's not 'the older you get, the sicker you get,' but 'the older you get, the healthier you've been.'" Now, that's the attitude to have.

The human body is an incredible product of natural selection and evolution. But evolution operates too slowly for the twenty-first-century individual. My goal is to extend human capabilities beyond what nature has provided so far. Wouldn't it be wonderful if we could end human diseases, improve human cognition and well-being, and have the ability to upgrade the biological features that are important to us?

From the time I started writing this book to now when you read this, thousands of studies have been published revealing new insights into health and disease. Novel theories about aging have been posited, some of which may change everything we thought we knew about a certain area of medicine. Though it's true that dogma can be hard to overturn, what's exciting about science is that it constantly endeavors to find the truth. When a new fact or discovery forces us to look and listen, we do. I have no doubt that in the future we will have much more than basic lifestyle tools to prevent disease and prolong life. Currently in rapid development, for example, are studies on therapeutic opportunities using various de-aging drugs and stem cell technology. Twenty years ago, we knew nothing about the human microbiome—the microbes that live within and on us and contribute to our health. Twenty years from now, we'll probably have another new area of medicine that doesn't yet exist. These are exciting times. The speed of our advances is like nothing the human species has ever experienced.

The science of autophagy may be just getting started in research circles, but the process has been around for billions of years—before we humans even emerged. Its scientific validity has already been shown in the populations of peoples and other animals I covered in the book. Future research will further shed light on this important topic, which plays into every area of medicine. Autophagy does not discriminate. Each one of us carries this vital process in our bodies no matter who we are or what genes we were born with. It's within you this instant, ready to be activated. But autophagy can tell the difference between a body that wants it turned on and one that leaves the Switch turned off. The strategies you've learned in this book are available to you; you just have to be willing to implement them in your own life. I urge you to do that. And please keep abreast of my work at https://betterhumans.org. On the link there to my Supercentenarian Study, you can see some of the incredible people I've had the pleasure of meeting (and collecting blood from) in search of their secrets to the fountain of youth. Their greatest legacy may be the discoveries we learn from them that benefit all of mankind.

Perhaps the best secret of all? This one comes courtesy of the late Clarence Matthews, whom I met shortly after his 110th birthday, and it will always stand the test of time: *Keep breathing*.

ACKNOWLEDGMENTS

This book has had a long and storied history, with many bright, enthusiastic people playing their part in its creation. I'd first like to thank Paul Carpenter for his encouragement and support, which included providing me with his lake cabin for the twelve months that it took me to research and write this book. And to my friend and colleague Parijata Mackey, who pushed me to discard dogma and question everything in cellular biology and medicine.

Anyone who has ever written a book knows that it takes a lively village from initially talking about it to getting it done and into the hands of readers who can benefit from the message. Kristin Loberg and I probably crossed paths unknowingly multiple times more than two decades ago while I was running a popular brewpub in Ithaca, New York, and she was a premed student at

ACKNOWLEDGMENTS

Cornell University. But it would take quite a while for us to have a conversation about this book—years after we'd both abandoned those pursuits and left Ithaca—and to map it all out, write a solid proposal, and eventually a manuscript. Thanks for being my collaborator and for introducing me to Bonnie Solow, my exceptional agent, whose patience, grace, wit, and publishing wisdom got me through the process. This book would not have been the same without your creative and editorial genius, as well as your leadership through and through.

To my editor, Jeremie Ruby-Strauss, and his ever-attentive assistant, Brita Lundberg: From the first day we spoke about the book and you shared your excitement, I knew you'd be the perfect fit to bring this important message to life on the page. It's been an absolute pleasure to work with you. And thanks to the rest of the publishing team at Simon & Schuster: Carolyn Reidy, Jon Karp, Jen Bergstrom, Aimée Bell, Jen Long, Eliza Hanson, Sally Marvin, Abby Zidle, Anne Jaconette, Anabel Jimenez, Lisa Litwack, John Vairo, Davina Mock, Caroline Pallotta, Allison Green, Christine Masters, and Kaitlyn Snowden. Thanks also to Celeste Phillips, who let me know where I needed to tone down my language lest I have a mad cow or nut come after me.

Finally, a special thanks to my mentors and friends George Church and David Sinclair—two giants in Harvard Medical School's genetics department—who persuaded me to write this book in order to share what I'd learned with others. Now let's spread the word to friends, family, and our health care givers that healthy aging and making it to 100 can be a choice!

NOTES

The following is a partial list of scientific papers and other references that you might find helpful in learning more about some of the ideas and concepts expressed in this book. I have cited the particular studies I mentioned here. If I had my wish, I'd cite every paper I've read on autophagy and life extension, but that would be impossible because the list would come to thousands of entries. At the least, these notes can open doors to further research and inquiry.

INTRODUCTION: THE SWITCH

1. GBD 2017 Diet Collaborators, "Health Effects of Dietary Risks in 195 Countries, 1990–2017: A Systematic Analysis

for the Global Burden of Disease Study 2017," *The Lancet* 393, no. 10184 (April 3, 2019): 1958–72.

2. Joana Araújo, Jianwen Cai, and June Stevens, "Prevalence of Optimal Metabolic Health in American Adults: National Health and Nutrition Examination Survey 2009–2016," *Metabolic Syndrome and Related Disorders* 17, no. 1 (February 2019): 46–52.

3. J. Graham Ruby, Kevin M. Wright, Kristin A. Rand, et al., "Estimates of the Heritability of Human Longevity Are Substantially Inflated Due to Assortative Mating," *Genetics* 210, no. 1 (November, 2018): 1109–24.

CHAPTER 1: EASTER ISLAND AND TRANSPLANT PATIENTS

1. Shelley X. Cao, Joseph M. Dhahbi, Patricia L. Mote, and Stephen R. Spindler, "Genomic Profiling of Short- and Long-Term Caloric Restriction Effects in the Liver of Aging Mice," *Proceedings of the National Academy of Sciences of the United States of America* 98, no. 19 (2001). You can access all of Spindler's research on his lab's website at https://biochemistry .ucr.edu/faculty/spindler/spindler_research_group.html.

2. For an overview of the story of rapamycin's discovery, see V. Koneti Rao, "Serendipity in Splendid Isolation: Rapamycin," *Blood* 127 (January 7, 2016): 5–6.

3. David M. Sabatini, Hediye Erdjument-Bromage, Mary Lui, et al., "RAFT1: A Mammalian Protein That Binds to FKBP12 in a Rapamycin-Dependent Fashion and Is Homologous to Yeast TORs," *Cell* 78, no. 1 (July 15, 1994): 35–43.

4. Anne N. Conner, "Could Rapamycin Help Humans Live Longer?," *The Scientist*, March 1, 2018.

5. Nicholas C. Barbet, Ulrich F. Schneider, Stephen B. Halliwell, et al., "TOR Controls Translation Initiation and Early G1 Progression in Yeast," *Molecular Biology of the Cell* 7, no. 1 (January 2017): 25–42.

6. For a review, see Charlotte Harrison, "Secrets of a Long Life," *Nature Reviews Drug Discovery* 8 (September 2009): 698–99.

7. David E. Harrison, Randy Strong, Zelton Dave Sharp, et al., "Rapamycin Fed Late in Life Extends Lifespan in Genetically Heterogeneous Mice," *Nature* 460, no. 7253 (July 16, 2009): 392–95.

8. Lan Ye, Anne L. Widlund, Carrie A. Sims, et al., "Rapamycin Doses Sufficient to Extend Lifespan Do Not Compromise Muscle Mitochondrial Content or Endurance," *Aging* 5, no. 7 (July 2013): 539–50.

9. John E. Wilkinson, Lisa Burmeister, Susan V. Brooks, et al., "Rapamycin Slows Aging in Mice," *Aging Cell* 11, no. 4 (August 2012): 675–82.

10. Chong Chen, Yu Liu, Yang Liu, and Pan Zheng, "mTOR Regulation and Therapeutic Rejuvenation of Aging Hematopoietic Stem Cells," *Science Signaling* 2, no. 98 (November 24, 2009): ra75.

11. Richard A. Miller, David E. Harrison, Clinton M. Astle, et al., "Rapamycin-Mediated Lifespan Increase in Mice Is Dose and Sex Dependent and Metabolically Distinct from Dietary Restriction," *Aging Cell* 13, no. 3 (June 2014): 468–77.

12. For a review of some of these dog studies, see Neil Savage,

"New Tricks from Old Dogs Join the Fight Against Ageing," *Nature* 552 (December 13, 2017): S57–S59.

13. Learn more about the Dog Aging Project at https://www .dogagingproject.org.

14. Mikhail V. Blagosklonny, "Aging and Immortality: Quasi-programmed Senescence and its Pharmacologic Inhibition," *Cell Cycle* 5, no. 18 (September 5, 2006): 2087–102.

CHAPTER 2: GARBAGE TRUCKS AND RECYCLING PLANTS

1. Vivien Marx, "Autophagy: Eat Thyself, Sustain Thyself," *Nature Methods* 12, no. 12 (December 2015): 1121–25.

2. For a great review of autophagy, see Susana Castro-Obregon, "The Discovery of Lysosomes and Autophagy," *Nature Education* 3, no. 9 (2010): 49.

3. Xiao Huan Liang, Saadiya Jackson, Matthew Seaman, et al., "Induction of Autophagy and Inhibition of Tumorigenesis by Beclin 1," *Nature* 402, no. 6762 (December 9, 1999): 672–76.

4. Robin Mathew, Vassiliki Karantza-Wadsworth, and Eileen White, "Role of Autophagy in Cancer," *Nature Reviews Cancer* 7, no. 12 (December 2007): 961–67.

CHAPTER 3: DWARFS AND MUTANTS

1. J. Graham Ruby, Kevin M. Wright, Kristin A. Rand, et al., "Estimates of the Heritability of Human Longevity Are Substantially Inflated Due to Assortative Mating," *Genetics* 210, no. 3 (November 2018): 1109–24.

2. Z. Laron, A. Pertzelan, and S. Mannheimer, "Genetic Pituitary Dwarfism with High Serum Concentration of Growth Hormone—A New Inborn Error of Metabolism?," *Israel Journal of Medical Sciences* 2, no. 2 (March–April 1966): 152–55. See also Zvi Laron, "Lessons from 50 Years of Study of Laron Syndrome," *Endocrine Practice* 21, no. 12 (December 2015): 1395–402.

3. Fernanda T. Gonçalves, Cintia Fridman, Emilia M. Pinto, et al., "The E180splice Mutation in the *GHR* Gene Causing Laron Syndrome: Witness of a Sephardic Jewish Exodus from the Iberian Peninsula to the New World?," *American Journal of Medical Genetics Part A* 164A, no. 5 (May 2014) 1204–08.

4. Jaime Guevara-Aguirre, Priya Balasubramanian, Marco Guevara-Aguirre, et al., "Growth Hormone Receptor Deficiency Is Associated with a Major Reduction in Pro-Aging Signaling, Cancer, and Diabetes in Humans," *Science Translational Medicine* 16, no. 3 (February 16, 2011): 70ra13.

5. O. Shevah and Z. Laron, "Patients with Congenital Deficiency of IGF-I Seem Protected from the Development of Malignancies: A Preliminary Report," *Growth Hormone & IGF Research* 17, no. 1 (February 2007): 54–57.

6. Kevin Flurkey, John Papacostantinou, Richard A. Miller, and David E. Harrison, "Lifespan Extension and Delayed Immune and Collagen Aging in Mutant Mice with Defects in Growth Hormone Production," *Proceedings of the National Academy of Sciences of the United States of America* 98, no. 12 (June 5, 2001): 6736–41.

7. Julie A. Mattison, Caradee Yael Wright, Roderick Terry Bronson, et al., "Studies of Aging in Ames Dwarf Mice: Effects

of Caloric Restriction," *Journal of the American Aging Association* 23, no. 1 (January 2000): 9–16. See also Andrzej Bartke and Reyhan Westbrook, "Metabolic Characteristics of Long-Lived Mice," *Frontiers in Genetics* 3 (December 13, 2012): 288.

8. Adam Gesing, Denise Wiesenborn, Andrew Do, et al., "A Long-Lived Mouse Lacking Both Growth Hormone and Growth Hormone Receptor: A New Animal Model for Aging Studies," *The Journals of Gerontology, Series A* 72, no. 8 (August 2017): 1054–61.

9. Gráinne S. Gorman, Patrick F. Chinnery, Salvatore DiMauro, et al., "Mitochondrial Diseases," *Nature Reviews Disease Primers* 2, article no. 16081 (October 20, 2016).

10. Alessandro Bitto, Chad Lerner, Claudio Torres, et al., "Long-Term IGF-1 Exposure Decreases Autophagy and Cell Viability," *PLoS ONE* 5, no. 9 (September 2010): e12592.

CHAPTER 4: OKINAWANS, MONKS, AND SEVENTH-DAY ADVENTISTS

1. Donald Craig Willcox, Bradley J. Willcox, Hidemi Todoriki, and Makoto Suzuki, "The Okinawan Diet: Health Implications of a Low-Calorie, Nutrient-Dense, Antioxidant-Rich Dietary Pattern Low in Glycemic Load," *Journal of the American College of Clinical Nutrition* 28 (suppl.) (August 2009): 500S–516S.

2. For more about the Okinawa Centenarian Study, see the Okinawa Research Center for Longevity Science, http://www.orcls.org.

3. C. M. McKay, Mary F. Crowell, and L. A. Maynard, "The Effect of Retarded Growth upon the Length of Life Span and

upon the Ultimate Body Size: One Figure," *The Journal of Nutrition* 10, no. 1 (July 1935): 63–79.

4. Richard Weindruch, Roy L. Walford, Suzanne Fligiel, and Donald Guthrie, "The Retardation of Aging in Mice by Dietary Restriction: Longevity, Cancer, Immunity, and Lifetime Energy Intake," *The Journal of Nutrition* 116, no. 4 (April 1986): 641–54.

5. Julie A. Mattison, Ricki J. Colman, T. Mark Beasley, et al., "Caloric Restriction Improves Health and Survival of Rhesus Monkeys," *Nature Communications* 8, article no. 14063 (January 17, 2017). See also Richard Conniff, "The Hunger Gains: Extreme Calorie-Restriction Diet Shows Anti-Aging Results," *Scientific American*, February 16, 2017, https://www.scientific american.com/article/the-hunger-gains-extreme-calorie -restriction-diet-shows-anti-aging-results/.

6. Min Wei, Sebastian Brandhorst, Mahshid Shelehchi, et al., "Fasting-mimicking Diet and Markers/Risk Factors for Aging, Diabetes, Cancer, and Cardiovascular Disease," *Science Translational Medicine* 9, no. 377 (February 15, 2017): 9.

7. See Calerie, https://calerie.duke.edu.

8. Emilie Leclerc, Allison Paulino Trevizol, Ruth B. Grigolon, et al., "The Effect of Caloric Restriction on Working Memory in Healthy Non-obese Adults," *CNS Spectrums* 10 (April 2017): 1–7.

9. James Rochon, Connie W. Bales, Eric Ravussin, et al., "Design and Conduct of the CALERIE Study: Comprehensive Assessment of the Long-Term Effects of Reducing Intake of Energy," *The Journals of Gerontology, Series A* 66 (January 2011): 97–108. See also Robert Roy Britt, "Live Longer: The One

Anti-Aging Trick That Works," Live Science, July 8, 2008, https://www.livescience.com/2666-live-longer-anti-aging -trick-works.html.

10. Edward P. Weiss, Dennis T. Villareal, Susan B. Racette, et al., "Caloric Restriction but Not Exercise-Induced Reductions in Fat Mass Decrease Plasma Triiodothyronine Concentrations: A Randomized Controlled Trial," *Rejuvenation Research* 11, no. 3 (June 2011): 605–09.

11. Edward P. Weiss, Stewart G. Albert, Dominic N. Reeds, et al., "Calorie Restriction and Matched Weight Loss from Exercise: Independent and Additive Effects on Glucoregulation and the Incretin System in Overweight Women and Men," *Diabetes Care* 38, no. 7 (July 2015): 1253–62.

12. Ana M. Andrade, Geoffrey W. Greene, and Kathleen J. Melanson, "Eating Slowly Led to Decreases in Energy Intake Within Meals in Healthy Women," *Journal of the American Dietetic Association* 108, no. 7 (July 2008): 1186–91.

13. Kaito Iwayama, Reiko Kurihara, Yoshiharu Nabekura, et al., "Exercise Increases 24-H Fat Oxidation Only When It Is Performed Before Breakfast," *EBioMedicine* 2, no. 12 (December 2012): 2003–09.

14. James D. LeCheminant, Ed Christenson, Bruce W. Bailey, and Larry A. Tucker, "Restricting Night-time Eating Reduces Daily Energy Intake in Healthy Young Men: A Short-Term Cross-over Study," *British Journal of Nutrition* 110, no. 11 (December 14, 2013): 2108–13.

15. Eric Robinson, Paul Aveyard, Amanda Daley, et al., "Eating Attentively: A Systematic Review and Meta-analysis of the Effect of Food Intake Memory and Awareness on Eating," *The*

American Journal of Clinical Nutrition 97, no. 4 (April 2013): 728–42.

16. Katerina O. Sarri, Nikolaos E. Tzanakis, Manolis K. Linardakis, et al., "Effects of Greek Orthodox Christian Church Fasting on Serum Lipids and Obesity," *BMC Public Health* 3 (May 16, 2003): 16.

17. Valter D. Longo and Mark P. Mattson, "Fasting: Molecular Mechanisms and Clinical Applications," *Cell Metabolism* 19, no. 2 (February 4, 2014): 181–92.

18. See Mark Mattson, "STEM-Talk Episode 7: Mark Mattson Talks About Benefits of Intermittent Fasting," Florida Institute for Human & Machine Cognition, April 12, 2016, https://www.ihmc.us/stemtalk/episode007/.

19. For Dr. Mattson's library of work, see his academic site at http://neuroscience.jhu.edu/research/faculty/57.

20. Stephen D. Anton, Keelin Moehl, William T. Donahoo, et al., "Flipping the Metabolic Switch: Understanding and Applying the Health Benefits of Fasting," *Obesity* 26, no. 2 (February 2016): 254–68.

21. Kelsey Gabel, Kristin K. Hoddy, Nicole Haggerty, et al., "Effects of 8-Hour Time Restricted Feeding on Body Weight and Metabolic Disease Risk Factors in Obese Adults: A Pilot Study," *Nutrition and Healthy Aging*, 4, no. 4 (June 15, 2018): 345–53.

22. Humaira Jamshed, Robbie A. Beyl, Deborah L. Della Manna, et al., "Early Time-Restricted Feeding Improves 24-Hour Glucose Levels and Affects Markers of the Circadian Clock, Aging, and Autophagy in Humans," *Nutrients* 11, no. 6 (June 2019): 1234.

23. For a general review, see Ioannis Delimaris, "Adverse Effects Associated with Protein Intake Above the Recommended Dietary Allowance for Adults," *ISRN Nutrition* (July 2013), article ID 126929.

24. Zeneng Wang, Nathalie Bergeron, Bruce S. Levison, et al., "Impact of Chronic Dietary Red Meat, White Meat, or Non-meat Protein on Trimethylamine N-Oxide Metabolism and Renal Excretion in Healthy Men and Women," *European Heart Journal* 40, no. 7 (February 14, 2019): 583–94.

25. Morgan E. Levine, Jorge A. Suarez, Sebastian Brandhorst, et al., "Low Protein Intake Is Associated with a Major Reduction in IGF-1, Cancer, and Overall Mortality in the 65 and Younger but Not Older Population," *Cell Metabolism* 19, no. 3 (March 4, 2014): 407–17.

26. Renata Micha, Jose E. Peñalvo, Frederick Cudhea, et al., "Association Between Dietary Factors and Mortality from Heart Disease, Stroke, and Type 2 Diabetes in the United States," *The Journal of the American Medical Association* 317, no. 9 (March 7, 2017): 912–24.

27. Yan Zheng, Yanping Li, Ambika Satija, et al., "Association of Changes in Red Meat Consumption with Total and Cause Specific Mortality Among US Women and Men: Two Prospective Cohort Studies," *The British Medical Journal* 365 (June 12, 2019), I2110. See also An Pan, Qi Sun, Adam M. Bernstein, et al., "Red Meat Consumption and Mortality: Results from 2 Prospective Cohort Studies," *Archives of Internal Medicine* 172, no. 7 (April 9, 2012): 555–63.

28. Heli E. K. Virtanen, Timo T. Koskinen, Sari Voutilainen, et al., "Intake of Different Dietary Proteins and Risk of Type 2

Diabetes in Men: The Kuopio Ischaemic Heart Disease Risk Factor Study," *British Journal of Nutrition* 117, no. 6 (March 2017): 882–93.

29. Alicja Wolk, Christos S. Mantzoros, Swen-Olof Andersson, et al., "Insulin-like Growth Factor 1 and Prostate Cancer Risk: A Population-Based, Case-Control Study," *Journal of the National Cancer Institute* 90, no. 12 (June 17, 1998): 911–15.

30. Simon Brooke-Taylor, Karen Dwyer, Keith Woodford, and Natalya Kost, "Systematic Review of the Gastrointestinal Effects of A1 Compared with A2 β-Casein," *Advances in Nutrition* 8, no. 5 (September 15, 2017): 739–48.

31. Yasuhiro Saito, Lewyn Li, Etienne Coyaud, et al., "LLGL2 Rescues Nutrient Stress by Promoting Leucine Uptake in ER+ Breast Cancer," *Nature* 569, no. 7775 (May 2019): 275–79.

CHAPTER 5: EPILEPTIC CHILDREN AND WORLD-CLASS CYCLISTS

1. Emory University Health Sciences Center, "Ketogenic Diet Prevents Seizures by Enhancing Brain Energy Production, Increasing Neuron Stability," ScienceDaily, November 15, 2005, www.sciencedaily.com/releases/2005/11/051114220938.htm.

2. Abbi R. Hernandez, Caesar M. Hernandez, Haila Campos, et al., "A Ketogenic Diet Improves Cognition and Has Biochemical Effects in Prefrontal Cortex That Are Dissociable from Hippocampus," *Frontiers in Aging Neuroscience* 10 (December 3, 2018): 391.

3. S. D. Phinney, B. R. Bistrian, W. J. Evans, et al., "The Human Metabolic Response to Chronic Ketosis without Caloric Restriction: Preservation of Submaximal Exercise Capability

with Reduced Carbohydrate Oxidation," *Metabolism* 32, no. 8 (August 1983): 769–76.

4. Brent C. Creighton, Parker Neil Hyde, Carl M. Maresh, et al., "Paradox of Hypercholesterolaemia in Highly Trained, Keto-Adapted Athletes," *BMJ Open Sport & Exercise Medicine* 4, no. 1 (October 2018).

5. Eric C. Westman, Justin Tondt, Emily Maguire, and William S. Yancy, Jr., "Implementing a Low-Carbohydrate, Ketogenic Diet to Manage Type 2 Diabetes Mellitus," *Expert Review of Endocrinology & Metabolism* 13, no. 5 (September 2018): 263–72. See also L. R. Saslow, S. Kim, J. J. Daubenmier, et al., "A Randomized Pilot Trial of a Moderate Carbohydrate Diet Compared to a Very Low Carbohydrate Diet in Overweight or Obese Individuals with Type 2 Diabetes Mellitus or Prediabetes," *PLoS ONE* 9, no. 4 (April 2014): e91027.

6. Gary Taubes, *Why We Get Fat: And What to Do About It* (New York: Knopf, 2010), 178.

7. Mahshid Dehghan, Andrew Mente, Xiaohe Zhang, et al., "Associations of Fats and Carbohydrate Intake with Cardiovascular Disease and Mortality in 18 Countries from Five Continents (PURE): A Prospective Cohort Study," *The Lancet* 390, no. 10107 (November 4, 2017): 2050–62.

8. Sarah J. Hallberg, Amy L. McKenzie, Paul T. Williams, et al., "Effectiveness and Safety of a Novel Care Model for the Management of Type 2 Diabetes at 1 Year: An Open-Label, Non-randomized, Controlled Study," *Diabetes Therapy* 9, no. 2 (April 2018): 583–612.

9. This quote is attributed to Eric Verdin, the president and CEO of the Buck Institute for Research on Aging and a coauthor of

a prominent paper on the ketogenic diet: John C. Newman, Anthony J. Covarrubias, Minghao Zhao, et al., "Ketogenic Diet Reduces Midlife Mortality and Improves Memory in Aging Mice," *Cell Metabolism* 26, no. 3 (September 5, 2017): 547–57.

10. Matthew K. Taylor, Debra K. Sullivan, Jonathan D. Mahnken, et al., "Feasibility and Efficacy Data from a Ketogenic Diet Intervention in Alzheimer's Disease," *Alzheimer's & Dementia* 4 (December 6, 2018): 28–36.

11. Michele G. Sullivan, "Fueling the Alzheimer's Brain with Fat," *Clinical Neurology News*, August 23, 2017, https://www.mdedge.com/clinicalneurologynews/article/145220/alzheimers-cognition/fueling-alzheimers-brain-fat.

12. Cinta Valls-Pedret, Aleix Sala-Vila, Mercè Serra-Mir, et al., "Mediterranean Diet and Age-Related Cognitive Decline: A Randomized Clinical Trial," *JAMA Internal Medicine* 175, no. 7 (July 2015): 1094–103.

13. John C. Newman, Anthony J. Covarrubias, Minghao Zhao, et al., "Ketogenic Diet Reduces Midlife Mortality and Improves Memory in Aging Mice," *Cell Metabolism* 26, no. 3 (September 5, 2017): 547–57. See also Megan N. Roberts, Marita A. Wallace, Alexey A. Tomilov, et al., "A Ketogenic Diet Extends Longevity and Healthspan in Adult Mice," *Cell Metabolism* 26, no. 3 (September 5, 2017): 539–46.

14. Roberts et al., "A Ketogenic Diet Extends Longevity and Healthspan in Adult Mice."

15. John C. Newman and Eric Verdin, "β-Hydroxybutyrate: A Signaling Metabolite," *Annual Review of Nutrition* 37 (August 2017): 51–76.

CHAPTER 6: CAVEMEN AND INDUSTRIALISTS

1. James V. Neel, Alan B. Weder, and Stevo Julius, "Type II Diabetes, Essential Hypertension, and Obesity as 'Syndromes of Impaired Genetic Homeostasis': The 'Thrifty Genotype' Hypothesis Enters the 21st Century," *Perspectives in Biology and Medicine* 42, no. 1 (Autumn 1998): 44–74.

2. This timeline is adapted from John Pickrell, "Timeline: Human Evolution," *New Scientist*, September 4, 2006, https://www .newscientist.com/article/dn9989-timeline-human-evolution/.

3. Vincent Balter, José Braga, Philippe Télouk and J. Francis Thackeray, "Evidence for Dietary Change but Not Landscape Use in South African Early Hominins," *Nature* 489, no. 7417 (September 27, 2012): 558–60.

4. Laure Schnabel, Emmanuelle Kesse-Guyot, Benjamin Allès, et al., "Association Between Ultraprocessed Food Consumption and Risk of Mortality Among Middle-Aged Adults in France," *JAMA Internal Medicine* 179, no. 4 (February 11, 2019): 490–98.

5. GBD 2017 Diet Collaborators, "Health Effects of Dietary Risks in 195 Countries, 1990–2017: A Systematic Analysis for the Global Burden of Disease Study 2017," *The Lancet* 393, no. 10184 (May 11, 2019): 1958–72.

6. Wolfgang Haak, Peter Forster, Barbara Bramanti, et al., "Ancient DNA from the first European Farmers in 7500-Year-Old Neolithic Sites," *Science* 310, no. 5750 (November 11, 2005): 1016–18.

7. Michael Gurven and Hillard Kaplan, "Longevity Among

Hunter-Gatherers: A Cross-Cultural Examination," *Population and Development Review* 33, no. 2 (June 2007): 321–65.

8. Michael P. Richards and Erik Trinkaus, "Isotopic Evidence for the Diets of European Neanderthals and Early Modern Humans," *Proceedings of the National Academy of Sciences of the United States of America* 106, no. 38 (September 22, 2009): 16034–39.

9. S. Boyd Eaton and Melvin Konner, "Paleolithic Nutrition—A Consideration of Its Nature and Current Implications," *The New England Journal of Medicine* 213, no. 5 (January 31, 1985): 283–89.

10. See "The Sugar Timeline," Hippocrates Health Institute, September 9, 2016, https://hippocratesinst.org/the-sugar-timeline. See also T. L. Cleave, *The Saccharine Disease: Conditions Caused by the Taking of Refined Carbohydrates, Such as Sugar and White Flour* (Bristol: John Wright & Sons, 1974).

11. See all of Loren Cordain's work at https://thepaleodiet.com/. See also Loren Cordain, S. Boyd Eaton, Anthony Sebastian, et al., "Origins and Evolution of the Western Diet: Health Implications for the 21st Century," *The American Journal of Clinical Nutrition* 81, no. 2 (February 2005): 341–54.

12. Da Li, Wu-Ping Sun, Shi-Sheng Zhou, et al., "Chronic Niacin Overload May Be Involved in the Increased Prevalence of Obesity in US Children," *World Journal of Gastroenterology* 16, no. 19 (May 21, 2010): 2378–87. See also Shi-Sheng Zhou, Da Li, Wu-Ping Sun, et al., "Nicotinamide Overload May Play a Role in the Development of Type 2 Diabetes," *World Journal of Gastroenterology* 15, no. 45 (December 7, 2009): 5674–84.

13. Ibid.

14. Jared Diamond, "The Worst Mistake in the History of the Human Race," *Discover*, May 1, 1987, 64–66.

15. Ibid.

16. Yuval Noah Harari, *Sapiens: A Brief History of Humankind* (New York: Harper, 2015), 91–92.

17. Yujin Lee, Dariush Mozaffarian, Stephen Sy, et al., "Cost-Effectiveness of Financial Incentives for Improving Diet and Health Through Medicare and Medicaid: A Microsimulation Study," *PLOS Medicine* 16, no. 3 (March 19, 2019): e1002761.

18. Gary Taubes, "Is Sugar Toxic?," *New York Times*, April 13, 2011.

19. Gary Taubes, *The Case Against Sugar* (New York: Knopf, 2016).

20. Robert Lustig, *Fat Chance: Beating the Odds Against Sugar, Processed Food, Obesity, and Disease* (New York: Hudson Street Press, 2012).

21. United States Department of Agriculture Economic Research Service, "Food Availability and Consumption," https://www.ers.usda.gov/data-products/ag-and-food-statistics-charting-the-essentials/food-availability-and-consumption/.

22. Emily E. Ventura, Jaimie N. Davis, and Michael I. Goran, "Sugar Content of Popular Sweetened Beverages Based on Objective Laboratory Analysis: Focus on Fructose Content," *Obesity* 19, no. 4 (April 2011): 868–74.

23. For a stunning review of chemicals that may cause obesity, see Bruce Blumberg, *The Obesogen Effect: Why We Eat Less and Exercise More but Still Struggle to Lose Weight* (New York: Grand Central, 2018).

CHAPTER 7: WALNUTS AND CORN-FED COWS

1. Penny M. Kris-Etherton, Thomas A. Pearson, Ying Wan, et al., "High-Monounsaturated Fatty Acid Diets Lower Both Plasma Cholesterol and Triacylglycerol Concentrations," *The American Journal of Clinical Nutrition* 70, no. 6 (December 1999): 1009–15.

2. Fumiaki Imamura, Renata Micha, Jason H. Y. Yu, et al., "Effects of Saturated Fat, Polyunsaturated Fat, Monounsaturated Fat, and Carbohydrate on Glucose-Insulin Homeostasis: A Systematic Review and Meta-analysis of Randomised Controlled Feeding Trials," *PLOS Medicine* 13, no. 7 (July 19, 2016): e1002087.

3. Maria Luz Fernandez and Kristy L. West, "Mechanisms by Which Dietary Fatty Acids Modulate Plasma Lipids," *The Journal of Nutrition* 135, no. 9 (September 2005): 2075–78. See also Olivia Gonçalves Leão Coelho, Bárbara Pereira da Silva, Daniela Mayumi Usuda Prado Rocha, et al., "Polyunsaturated Fatty Acids and Type 2 Diabetes: Impact on the Glycemic Control Mechanism," *Critical Reviews in Food Science and Nutrition* 57, no. 17 (November 22, 2017): 3614–19.

4. James V. Pottala, Kristine Yaffe, Jennifer G. Robinson, et al., "Higher RBC EPA + DHA Corresponds with Larger Total Brain and Hippocampal Volumes," *Neurology* 82, no. 5 (February 4, 2014): 435–42.

5. Z. S. Tan, W. S. Harris, A. S. Beiser, et al., "Red Blood Cell ω-3 Fatty Acid Levels and Markers of Accelerated Brain Aging," *Neurology* 78, no. 9 (February 28, 2012): 658–64.

6. See Framingham Heart Study, https://www.framinghamheart study.org.

7. Éric Dewailly, Carole Blanchet, Simone Lemieux, et al., "n-3 Fatty Acids and Cardiovascular Disease Risk Factors among the Inuit of Nunavik," *The American Journal of Clinical Nutrition* 74, no. 4 (October 2001): 464–73.

8. See Patricia Gadsby and Leon Steele, "The Inuit Paradox," *Discover*, October 1, 2004.

9. Cynthia A. Daley, Amber Abbott, Patrick S. Doyle, et al., "A Review of Fatty Acid Profiles and Antioxidant Content in Grass-Fed and Grain-Fed Beef," *Nutrition Journal* 9, no. 10 (March 2010).

10. Éric Dewailly was a Canadian epidemiologist who studied the Inuit paradox throughout his career, as well as the effects of contaminants on the environment in the Arctic. He is credited for calling omega-3 polyunsaturated fats a "natural aspirin" to dampen inflammatory processes.

11. See Bodil Schmidt-Nielsen, *August and Marie Krogh: Lives in Science* (New York: Springer, 1995).

12. Hans Olaf Bang and Jørn Dyerberg, "Lipid Metabolism and Ischemic Heart Disease in Greenland Eskimos," in *Advances in Nutritional Research*, edited by H. H. Draper (New York: Springer Science+Business Media, 1980), 1–22.

13. Cynthia A. Daley, Amber Abbott, Patrick S. Doyle, et al., "A Review of Fatty Acid Profiles and Antioxidant Content in Grass-Fed and Grain-Fed Beef," *Nutrition Journal* 9, no. 10 (March 2010).

14. Christopher E. Ramsden, Daisy Zamora, Boonseng Leelar-

thaepin, et al., "Use of Dietary Linoleic Acid for Secondary Prevention of Coronary Heart Disease and Death: Evaluation of Recovered Data from the Sydney Diet Heart Study and Updated Meta-analysis," *The British Medical Journal* 346 (February 4, 2013): e8707.

15. Michel de Lorgeril, Patricia Salen, Jean-Louis Martin, et al., "Mediterranean Diet, Traditional Risk Factors, and the Rate of Cardiovascular Complications After Myocardial Infarction: Final Report of the Lyon Diet Heart Study," *Circulation* 99, no. 6 (February 16, 1999): 779–85.

16. Frank M. Sacks, Alice H. Lichtenstein, Jason H. Y. Yu, et al., "Dietary Fats and Cardiovascular Disease: A Presidential Advisory from the American Heart Association," *Circulation* 136, no. 3 (2017): e1–e23.

17. Artemis P. Simopoulos, "The Mediterranean Diets: What Is So Special About the Diet of Greece? The Scientific Evidence," *The Journal of Nutrition* 131, no. 11 (suppl.) (November 2001): 3065S–73S.

18. Ramón Estruch, Emilio Ros, Jordi Salas-Salvadó, et al., "Primary Prevention of Cardiovascular Disease with a Mediterranean Diet," *The New England Journal of Medicine* 368, no. 14 (April 4, 2013): 1279–90.

19. Ramón Estruch, Emilio Ros, Jordi Salas-Salvadó, et al., "Primary Prevention of Cardiovascular Disease with a Mediterranean Diet Supplemented with Extra-Virgin Olive Oil or Nuts," *The New England Journal of Medicine* 378, no. 25 (June 21, 2018): e34.

20. Michelle Luciano, Janie Corley, Simon R. Cox, et al.,

"Mediterranean-Type Diet and Brain Structural Change from 73 to 76 Years in a Scottish Cohort," *Neurology* 88, no. 5 (January 31, 2017): 449–55.

21. Gretchen Benson, Raquel Franzini Pereira, and Jackie L. Boucher, "Rationale for the Use of a Mediterranean Diet in Diabetes Management," *Diabetes Spectrum* 24, no. 1 (February 2011): 36–40.

22. Shusuke Yagi, Daiju Fukuda, Ken-ichi Aihara, et al., "n-3 Polyunsaturated Fatty Acids: Promising Nutrients for Preventing Cardiovascular Disease," *Journal of Atherosclerosis and Thrombosis* 24, no. 10 (October 1, 2017): 999–1010.

23. Narinder Kaur, Vishal Chugh, and Anil K. Gupta, "Essential Fatty Acids as Functional Components of Foods—A Review," *Journal of Food Science and Technology* 51, no. 10 (October 2014): 2289–303.

24. Asmaa S. Abdelhamid, Tracey J. Brown, Julii S. Brainard, et al., "Omega-3 Fatty Acids for the Primary and Secondary Prevention of Cardiovascular Disease," Cochran Database of Systematic Reviews, November 30, 2018.

CHAPTER 8: WHALES, RODENTS, AND SMOKERS

1. For more, see https://www.afsc.noaa.gov/nmml/library/.

2. John C. George, Jeffrey Bada, Judith Zeh, et al., "Age and Growth Estimates of Bowhead Whales (*Balaena mysticetus*) via Aspartic Acid Racemization," *Canadian Journal of Zoology* 77, no. 4 (September 1999): 571–80. See also Cheryl Rosa, J. Craig George, Judith Zeh, et al., "Update on Age Estimation of Bowhead Whales (*Balaena mysticetus*) Using Aspartic

Acid Racemization," n.d., http://www.north-slope.org/assets/images/uploads/SC-56-BRG6_ROSA.pdf.

3. Arkadi F. Prokopov, "Theoretical Paper: Exploring Overlooked Natural Mitochondria-Rejuvenative Intervention: The Puzzle of Bowhead Whales and Naked Mole Rats," *Rejuvenation Research* 10, no. 4 (December 2007): 543–60. See also L. Michael Philo, Emmett B. Shotts Jr., and John C. George, "Morbidity and Mortality," in *The Bowhead Whale*, edited by John J. Burns, J. Jerome Montague, and Cleveland J. Cowles (Lawrence, KS: Society for Marine Mammalogy, 1993), 275–312.

4. For a review of her work and that of others, see J. Graham Ruby, Megan Smith, and Rochelle Buffenstein, "Naked Mole-Rat Mortality Rates Defy Gompertzian Laws by Not Increasing with Age," eLife 7 (January 24, 2018): e31157.

5. S. Zhao, L. Lin, G. Kan, et al., "High Autophagy in the Naked Mole Rat May Play a Significant Role in Maintaining Good Health," *Cellular Physiology and Biochemistry* 33, no. 2 (2014): 321–32.

6. Edward J. Calabrese and Linda A. Baldwin, "Hormesis: U-shaped Dose Responses and Their Centrality in Toxicology," *Trends in Pharmacological Science* 22, no. 6 (June 2001): 285–91.

7. Michael Roerecke and Jürgen Rehm, "The Cardioprotective Association of Average Alcohol Consumption and Ischaemic Heart Disease: A Systematic Review and Meta-analysis," *Addiction* 107, no. 7 (July 2012): 1246–60.

8. Edward J. Calabrese and Mark P. Mattson, "How Does Hormesis Impact Biology, Toxicology, and Medicine?," *NPJ Aging and Mechanisms of Disease* 3, article no. 13 (2017).

9. Edward J. Calabrese and Linda A. Baldwin, "Hormesis as a Biological Hypothesis," *Environmental Health Perspectives* 106 (suppl. 1) (February 1998): 357–62.

10. Gary E. Goodman, Mark D. Thornquist, John Balmes, et al., "The Beta-Carotene and Retinol Efficacy Trial: Incidence of Lung Cancer and Cardiovascular Disease Mortality During 6-year Follow-up After Stopping β-carotene and Retinol Supplements," *Journal of the National Cancer Institute* 96, no. 23 (December 2004): 1743–50.

11. See "Welcome to the ATBA Study Web Site," National Cancer Institute, https://atbcstudy.cancer.gov.

12. Scott M. Lippman, Eric A. Klein, Phyllis J. Goodman, et al., "Effect of Selenium and Vitamin E on Risk of Prostate Cancer and Other Cancers: The Selenium and Vitamin E Cancer Prevention Trial (SELECT)," *The Journal of the American Medical Association* 30, no. 1 (January 7, 2009): 39–51.

13. Eric A. Klein, Ian M. Thompson, Catherine M. Tangen, et al., "Vitamin E and the Risk of Prostate Cancer: The Selenium and Vitamin E Cancer Prevention Trial (SELECT)," *The Journal of the American Medical Association* 306, no. 14 (October 12, 2011): 1549–56.

14. Volkan I. Sayin, Mohamed X. Ibraham, Erik Larsson, et al., "Antioxidants Accelerate Lung Cancer Progression in Mice," *Science Translational Medicine* 6, no. 221 (January 29, 2014): 221ra15.

15. Kristell Le Gal, Mohamed X. Ibrahim, Clotilde Wiel, et al., "Antioxidants Can Increase Melanoma Metastasis in Mice," *Science Translational Medicine* 7, no. 308 (October 7, 2015): 308re8.

16. Ewen Callaway, "How Elephants Avoid Cancer," *Nature*, October 8, 2015, https://www.nature.com/news/how-elephants-avoid-cancer-1.18534. See also Lisa M. Abegglen, Aleah F. Caulin, Ashley Chan, et al., "Potential Mechanisms for Cancer Resistance in Elephants and Comparative Cellular Response to DNA Damage in Humans," *The Journal of the American Medical Association* 314, no. 17 (November 3, 2015): 1850–60.

CHAPTER 9: FINGER PRICKS AND GROCERY LISTS

1. Congcong He, Michael E. Bassik, Viviana Moresi, et al., "Exercise-Induced BCL2-Regulated Autophagy Is Required for Muscle Glucose Homeostasis," *Nature* 481, no. 7382 (January 26, 2012): 511–15.
2. Xiao Huan Liang, Saadiya Jackson, Matthew Seaman, et al., "Induction of Autophagy and Inhibition of Tumorigenesis by Beclin 1," *Nature* 402, no. 6762 (December 9, 1999): 672–76.
3. Alicia Meléndez and Beth Levine and A. Meléndez, "Autophagy in *C. elegans*," WormBook, August 24, 2009, http://www.wormbook.org/chapters/www_autophagy/autophagy.html.
4. Y. He, Germaine G. Cornelissen-Guillaume, Junyun He, et al., "Circadian Rhythm of Autophagy Proteins in Hippocampus Is Blunted by Sleep Fragmentation," *Chronobiology International* 33, no. 5 (2016): 553–60.
5. See National Sleep Foundation, htps://www.sleepfoundation.org.

IMAGE CREDITS

Page 21: Ian Sewell via Wikimedia Commons

Page 37: Emma Farmer via Wikimedia Commons

Page 40: *Elsevier Science*, 23/6, Eva Dazert and Michael N. Hall, mTOR signaling in disease, 746, Copyright 2011, with permission from Elsevier

Page 53: Courtesy of the National Human Genome Research Institute, genome.gov

Page 55: Kashmiri, based on earlier work by Domaina, via Wikimedia Commons

Page 65: iStock.com/Eriklam

Page 131: CartoonStock.com

Page 147: Radiogenic via Wikimedia Commons

Page 194: Chris huh (converted by King of Hearts) via Wikimedia Commons

Page 198: Courtesy of the author

Page 206: Eric Gaba (User: Sting) via Wikimedia Commons

INDEX

INDEX